Table of Contents

OVER 40 AND STILL HOT!

It's time to get your sexy back

Contact: help@over40stillhot.com

An Ode to ALL of Us fabulous ladies Who are Over 40 & Still Hot

I know I'm not young
However, I know I'm not dead.

But I must admit
I look at my birthdays with dread.

How did this happen
I really want to know.

If aging is for others
Why must I ask, where did my body go?

True, I've noticed some lines
Maybe a few extra pounds.

But that doesn't mean I'm ready
To bury my head in the ground.

I'm better than those 20-somethings
30-somethings too.

Although no offense
If that happens to be you.

So my boobs aren't where they used to be
And maybe my belly isn't as flat.

But that doesn't mean
I can't be all that.

Hotness isn't about having the perfect body
Or most attractive face.

Because if that's all it was
No one would ever win that race.

Every age has its issues
With body flaws and things to hide.

That's why we all need to learn
It's not about the destination; it's really about the ride.

Living your life with passion
Offering each other more grace.

Learning to love who you are
Waking up with a smile on your face.

Being over 40 is really the best.
I'm stronger. More confident. I'm reaching for my peak.

There is no way in the world
I could ever be labeled as weak.

Over 40 is my time to shine
Show the world what I've got.

So yes, I may be over 40
But look out, because I know I'm STILL hot!

Disclaimer

Always consult with your physician before beginning any exercise or weight-loss program. The information included in this eBook and website is not intended to substitute for a medical consultation or replace your healthcare professional. We make no representations or warranties concerning any usage of the information offered here and will not be liable for any direct, indirect, consequential, special, exemplary or other losses or damages that may result. Reliance on any information appearing on this site or from me is strictly at your own risk.

The author, company, affiliates, or any other parties involved in the creation or promotion of our products are not responsible for any injuries or health conditions that may result from advice, opinions, and programs represented in this website or any of our eBooks, training programs or other products. The information included in this eBook and in the training program are the opinions of the author. If you choose to follow any Over 40 and Still Hot fitness and wellness program without consulting your physician, you are doing so at your own risk.

We claim no responsibility for any injuries you might sustain. Exercise diagrams and detailed descriptions are included to give you the information needed to be able to perform the exercise with proper form. However, it is your responsibility to warm up properly, determine the correct amount of weight to use, perform each movement correctly, and ultimately decide whether you are capable of performing the exercise/workout without sustaining injury.

As with any exercise program, if at any point during your workout you begin to feel faint, dizzy, have physical discomfort or pain, you should stop immediately and consult a physician.

Hallelujah - You Made It!

You made it past the big 4-0. Not as scary as it seems to be older than 39 is it?

Seriously, what is the big deal about being over 40? Being over 40 is fabulous!

By the time you hit your 40s, you've probably hit a few bumps in the road. Well, maybe more than a few. The end result? You've got more confidence, don't care as much as what people think, and have a good grip on who it is you are.

And if that's not fabulous, I don't know what is.

So what if some things aren't quite the same in your body as they used to be? Would you ***really*** want to go back to your life when you were in your 20s just because your tummy was flatter and you didn't have the so called "old lady" arm waggle? No way!

You can still have a great looking body AND all the confidence that being over 40 brings. What could be better than that?

This book is all about getting your body and your sexy back. Being over 40 means that you've probably realized that not everything in life is perfect and that means your body too. But things that are imperfect can often times be the most beautiful. And no one has the perfect body, no matter what their age. But that doesn't mean that you can't look and feel fabulous. You absolutely can. You've just got to make the commitment to yourself.

It's time to get your sexy back. Let's get started!!!

Whether you are just getting started by working out for the first time, getting back into it after some off-months (or years), or you have been active for your entire life and you're just looking for something new and different, welcome to the Over 40 and Still Hot community! I truly mean that. Your commitment to your body, your mind, and your spirit and taking it to the next level is what it's all about. The reward is a stronger, sleeker, happier, and of course, sexier YOU!

I know it's not always easy to take time out for yourself. As women, we all seem to be pulled in different directions. Spouses, significant others, kids, jobs, activities as well as friends and family obligations can keep us hopping around. In fact, you might even be wondering how to fit this program into your busy schedule.

I've been involved in fitness for over 20 years and I have been a fitness instructor for the past 6. I work solely with women. And over the years I came to the realization that somewhere around the 40 mark, we start to lose our sexy.

It's not because you're busy. That's just a piece of the puzzle. Rather, it's because our physical bodies are changing too. I mean, who hasn't woken up and looked in the mirror and discovered cellulite or back fat where there wasn't any the day before? Not to mention the changes in our skin texture and tone, a few new aches and pains, and the wrinkles that start spreading around eyes, lips and neck.

However, fitting in a fitness and wellness regime will really help you to feel better, look better, sleep better, and deal with all the crazy things you have going on.

Finding new ways to keep yourself motivated, working the muscles in different ways, toning up those trouble spots and mixing up your diet are just some of the things that you'll learn about while reading this eBook. Most importantly, just simply by taking the time to read this eBook, whether you implement everything or not (although I hope that you do!), means that you are taking the steps to living an active, dynamic life in a way that honors you and your body.

Over 40 and Still Hot is designed to be a total fitness system. It offers challenging and effective exercises that will keep you engaged and motivated so you can get the results that you want. Trust me; you're not alone in having your trouble spots. We all have them. Especially once we start getting around the age of 40, give or take a few years of course. The arms start to jiggle; the belly pooches, the butt drops and love handles start to develop. And if you've had any children, well, this tends to speed the process up a little bit. Rest assured, though, it happens to all of us.

Let's face it though. You're getting older. And really, what's wrong with that? Nothing! As you get older, you mature, meaning you're way more at peace with who and what you are. I'm in my 40's and I'm loving it.

Of course, that still doesn't mean that you don't want to improve a few things, right?

Despite what you may have read or heard, at the end of the day there really is nothing that can stop the aging process. BUT, and that's a really big but (no pun intended), there are LOTS of things you can do to start to take control of the process. You CAN tone up your body and decrease those trouble spots so they are a whole lot less noticeable. You CAN eat healthier and drink more water so that you look healthy, feel healthy and have skin that glows. You CAN do things to eliminate your stress and learn to sleep more which helps further by making you look more rested and keeping your metabolism revved. Most of all, it's about learning and doing things that change things up and keep your body, as well as your brain, feeling and looking at its peak.

One of the best ways to do this is to find workouts that not only fit into your schedule, but also challenge you both mentally AND physically.

Getting to that next level of fitness isn’t easy, regardless of where you are at right now.

Actually, I want to dispel a myth. I believe that fitness is easy. All that you need to do is move more and eat less. However, it’s making the time for it and then actually doing it that makes achieving true fitness seem so hard.

Don’t think that it’s just you; it’s tough for everyone. It takes time, dedication, and commitment. Trust me, you may see a woman who looks phenomenal and effortlessly put together. If you’re like a lot of women, you wonder how she can look so much better than you. But you’re just looking at the results of her hard work: she’s had to find the time for herself. Somehow, she managed to fit herself into her busy schedule. If she can do it, so can you. Don’t make the excuse that you’re busy; we’re all busy. If you don't make the effort to take time for yourself and take care of yourself, you can't expect anyone else to do it either.

In this eBook, you're going to find a lot of information on general health, nutrition, and of course, exercises that are going to get you results and help minimize those trouble spots.

Now, you can pick and choose what you want out of the information that I'm providing. You may decide you just want to work on your diet. Or maybe, you're just looking for some workouts to get you started.

But that's doing yourself a disservice.

Yes, if you just watch your diet, you'll probably lose some pounds. And yes, if you just concentrate on the workouts you'll probably see some changes in how you look. Even if you decide that you don't feel like doing your workouts once or twice a week you'll probably see changes. But those results will be greatly diminished if you're only doing part of what I'm recommending.

To get the best results, you need to incorporate all of the elements in this eBook.

When you change your diet and incorporate all elements of the workouts you'll see your results increase exponentially.

In regards to the workouts, a good rule of thumb to follow is that if it feels easy, you aren't working out at your maximum level. You need to push yourself and work hard. I'm not talking about working to the point of pain, or injuring yourself. I want you to work just to the point where you know you've worked.

Work to your max; don't do it halfway. Going all out, with the best of what you have that day, is the only way you're going to see results. That's what you are looking for after all.

So demand only the best from yourself. Give 100% of whatever you have that day. Trust me; it changes every day depending on sleep, stress, nutrition and a whole host of other things. Some days you'll have tons of energy and others you may not be able to go at it quite as hard. Just do your best to give 100% of what you can on that particular day. It's only when you do that can you expect body and life-changing results.

Here's to your success and getting your body back!

xoxo

Debby

GETTING YOUR GROVE ON

HOW DID I GET HERE?

Never thought it would happen to you, huh? Other people get old, but that's not supposed to happen to you. I didn't think it would happen to me either. Unfortunately, I'm sad to say, none of us are immune.

Have you ever wondered why there are all these changes going on in your body as you age? It's not just you, I promise. It's all women.

We all find ourselves asking the same questions. Why do we all start to get a little droopy and saggy as we get older? Why does the fat seem to shift around? Why does it all seem to happen at, or right around, the decade mark? It's more than just a crappy birthday present.

Turns out, our bodies are constantly evolving. That's because many of the living cells in our bodies are replaced every 7 to 10 years. That includes fat cells, which are replaced at a rate of 10% a year.

That's part of why it seems like you wake up with a whole new body on every big birthday. I know, I know, it's not the gift you really wanted. I've personally tried to put an aging moratorium on my house, but that doesn't seem to be working. But when you think about it and wrap your head around it, it just logically makes sense that your body won't remain exactly the same, right? It's constantly evolving.

Making things worse, our metabolism starts to slow down too once we get past 30. Plus, the effects of gravity start to take their toll. The result? By the time you hit your 40s, you might not be quite as pleased with your new body as you were with the old one. That's why it's important to eat right and work out. Because when you work out and eat right, your body is less likely to show the effects of aging. This helps you to stay as close to your original body as you possibly can.

OK, I have to be real here and give you full disclosure. Why? Because it's my commitment to always be honest with you, even though you might not like what I have to say.

Here it is: I can't promise you'll get back the body of your 20s. I'm not saying you won't look fantastic or that you can't be in even better shape. But to say that you'll get the body of a 20-something-year-old again? Probably not gonna happen. No one can promise you that. And if they do, run for the hills.

So what if you don't get exactly back to where you once were? You can definitely still have a great body at any age. I'm talking about one where you're not embarrassed to go sleeveless. Or wear shorts. Or even a bathing suit. A body you feel good about. One that makes you feel like the confident, hot and sexy woman you are inside. Really.

It comes down to making the decision about what you want.

Now, there is no diet or exercise program in the world, regardless of what it claims, that can magically give you a perfect body. You can't spot reduce (which means only losing weight in your arms or your belly by working directly on them). But with the right nutrition and proper exercise, you can tone and firm up all over so that those problem spots aren't quite as noticeable and don't seem as big of a problem.

Look, I'm proud to say I'm in my 40s. At my age I can still wear shorts and go sleeveless. Heck, I'll still go out in public in a bikini too. I may not look like a movie star in it, but I'm not embarrassed to be seen either.

I'm not saying this to brag; I'm telling you this because I'm really just like you. I have body issues and family genetics that I'm fighting against too. The women in my family tend to be short with muscular thighs, flat butts and the uncanny ability to gain most of our weight in our midsection. We're the classic apple shape, but with the added bonus of curvy stumpy legs thrown in just for fun and frustrating shopping experiences.

It's something that I battle every day. Maybe battle is too strong a word, but it's something I choose to work on every day. And let me be clear about that, it is a choice. I make the decision to eat right and workout. Trust me; I'm not always in the mood. There are some days

I just want to be a slug and eat junk food all day.

I'm not going to lie to you and say I never give in to that urge. Of course I do! I'm human after all. However, I know what will happen if I give in to that urge too often. So instead, I stay focused on my goal. I don't want to turn back the hands of time, but I want look as good as I can at my age for as long as I possibly can.

I don't follow some crazy diet or do the latest and greatest workout craze. I watch my calories, eat a balanced diet and work out 6 days a week doing workouts just like ones I recommend in this book and on my website www.Over40StillHot.com. It's the formula I follow and it works for me. It works for my clients. And yes, it will work for you too.

That's why I can honestly tell you, at the end of the day, your lifestyle, mindset and activity level ultimately WILL help dictate how your body ages. The more you keep your body active and feed it correctly, not only will you feel younger, you'll look younger too.

If I can do it, you can do it too.

So let's get started!

SETTING GOALS

No matter where you're starting from, to get to the next level of fitness and wellness, you first need to figure out what that next level is for you. In other words, you need to determine your destination in order to get the proper directions. This is really important so don't brush this part off.

Think about it like driving a car. How are you supposed to get somewhere if you don't know where you're going in the first place? So get out the pen and pad of paper, iPad or whatever. It's time to figure out where you want to be and what you define as true fitness and wellness.

Take some time and think this over. But also make sure that you don't sweat it either. This isn't supposed to be an exam and no one is going to grade you. In fact, your answers probably won't match anyone else's answers. It's a very personal thing. This is just something to answer for yourself so that you get a baseline of where you're at. Think about these questions:

- What area of my fitness am I the most happy with?
  - *Example: I drink 8 glasses of water a day, I do yoga occasionally, I eat my 5 fruits and veggies, I take a multi vitamin, I sleep 7-8 hours a night, I walk the dog every day, I can run XXX miles.*

- What area of my fitness would I like to see the most improvement?
  - *Example: I want to drink 8 glasses of water a day, I want toned arms, I want to walk/run a 5k (or a marathon!), and I want to eat more vegetables.*

- What goal can I set to prove TO MYSELF that I have improved?
  - *Example: I completed a race, I lost XXX pounds, I lost XXX*

inches, and I no longer eat potato chips every day.

- What am I willing to do to get there?
    - *Example: I am willing to get up early, I am willing to work out 5 days a week, I am willing to buy more organic foods, I am willing to workout with a friend, etc.*
- What are you willing to give up in order to meet those goals?
    - *Example: I am willing to give up some of my clothing money so I can buy workout clothes, I am willing to give up candy, I am willing to give up sleeping in on weekends, etc.*

Look at those questions and think about them. In other words, take stock of your personal fitness. Think of where you are right now and where you want to be. Don't think of it in just short term goals like where you want to be tomorrow or a month from now. That's fine, but you also need to look a year, two years, even 20 years down the road.

I once had a woman in my boot camp who took my class five days a week for 2 months. She lost weight, multiple inches, and looked fantastic. At the end of two months she came up to me to say thank you for helping her get her body back. I said you're welcome and how proud I was of her and how happy I was that she reached her goals. As I told her I was looking forward to seeing her at the next class, she gave me a strange look and said, "Why? I'm in shape now. I don't need to come back and workout anymore."

Oh, how I wish it was that easy! Do all the hard work once in our lives and reap the rewards for the rest of our lives. We'd all look fabulous all the time then, right?

But a life of fitness and true wellness is a never ending process. It's just like any personal relationship that you value. You have to be consistent and work at it all the time. Once you stop, all of your hard work will eventually go away and you will end up right back where you started. That's why you need to think of wellness as a lifelong commitment to yourself.

It's just like anything else in life. If you want something, you have to do more than just think about it. You have to take action and work for it.

But first, you have to identify your goals and what it is that you really want.

When you're thinking about your goals, think about them in larger terms. Not just what you weigh, what size you wear, or how fast and far you can run. Although that's part of it, you need to stay focused on the big picture.

Here are a couple of examples for you. Don't worry about whether or not you identify with them. They're just here to get you started.

- Molly does a yoga CD program several times a week. She's has gotten more flexible and feels good. However, she gets breathless after going up several flights of stairs. She'd like to to improve her cardio fitness. She dreams of someday completing her first 5k race.

- Sarah is a couch potato. While she used to work out a bit when she was younger, she hasn't done anything in years. Not to mention, she has a bit of an addiction to junk food and likes her beer and wine. Now, she has at least 20 pounds to lose. Susan's goal? To work on her overall fitness, improve her diet and drop at least one full size.

- Jane's a great runner and has completed several races including a marathon. However, she has no upper body strength and is embarrassed by her flabby arms. Her goal? Being able to go sleeveless without feeling self-conscious.

- Alex goes to the gym three times a week but she spends more time talking than she does working out when she's there. She's in OK shape. She's got a stressful job and three kids. To get through it all, she's become addicted to coffee and has five big cups a day. All that caffeine makes it hard for her to sleep at night so she's always tired. Her goal? Cut down the caffeine to two cups a day and make her time at the gym more meaningful to help her manage her stress.

So let's break it down.

1. What area of my fitness am I the most happy with?

   Think about it this way. What do you see as your strengths? What do you know that you are doing right? Are you the cardio queen? Even if you don't work out, do you eat right or even OK? Do you get enough sleep? Are you always up for trying something new? Are you religious in your dedication to your workouts? Do you limit your caffeine? Avoid processed foods? These are all strengths. Write them down, no matter how big or small. Be proud of all the great things that you do to keep your body strong. Even if you can only think of one thing to start, including buying this eBook, that's great! Celebrate that you're taking a step forward. As long as you are moving forward, that's all that counts.

2. What area of my fitness would I like to see the most improvement?

   Here's the part that most of us could write pages about. Basically, the question should be: where do you think that you need a kick in the pants? Areas you know that you need a little help with.

   Go ahead and go crazy. Write them all down; everything, both big and small. Then I want you to prioritize them in order of importance to you. Because here's the kicker: You're going to limit your areas of improvement to only two things.

   Yes, you read that right. Just two. I don't care if you're a fitness rock star or simply an overachiever who hates failure - you just get two.

   Why only two? Because anything you write down here requires changing your habits. I don't care who you are or what you've accomplished, changing a habit, one that you've probably had for years, is never easy. Giving up just one thing or making one small change can be very hard. Trying to change all of your habits on the list and doing it all at once can seem daunting and overwhelming. Trying to do everything all at once is just crazy and just sets us up for failure. So stick to two.

Trust me, once you've successfully accomplished changing two habits, feel free to go back and work on the next two. This isn't a once and done thing where you only get two and you have to forget about the rest of your list. This is a process. The important thing is that you keep moving forward.

Once you've identified the two goals that you want to start working on first, I want you to go back and answer the following:

- What goal can I set to prove TO MYSELF that I have improved?

- What are you willing to do to get there?
- What are you willing to give up to meet that goal?

Try to remember that that this isn't a competition against anyone; don't use anyone else as a benchmark. We each have different strengths and weaknesses. What one of us loves to do, another may try it out and hate it. That's OK; that's what makes the world go round. Face it: you're not going to love everything. So pick something that works for YOU.

Here's a great worksheet to help you get started. This isn't homework, nor is there a test. It's just to give you a baseline of where you are at right now as well as where you want to be and how you're going to get there.

If you want to go back and do this again, I've also included an extra copy at the end of the book.

Setting My Fitness Goals Worksheet

- What areas of my fitness am I most happy with?

- What area of my fitness would I like to see the most improvement? List them all.

- What are the top two areas that I would like to work on first?

- What goal can I set for myself to prove TO MYSELF that I have improved?

- What am I willing to do to get there?

- What are you willing to give up in order to meet your goals?

Congratulations!

You now have the start of a plan!!!

CRAP! DO I HAVE TO DO EVERY DAY?

I'm often asked, especially by women who are just getting started, how many times per week you should workout. Especially from women who are trying to lose weight.

Maybe you're already working out, but you're not quite getting the results you want and you're wondering what the heck you really need to do to jump start your workouts.

I have to be honest and say that I always hesitate on this one. The best answer is, "It depends."

If you are just starting out, you need to start out at a level that you feel comfortable with so that you'll be able to stick with it. That doesn't mean you should go full force five days a week. It might be two to three days of more intense workouts along with 2-3 days of easier ones. You can always add more intense days when you're ready. Consistency is the key to getting fit.

However, your goal should be at least five workouts a week with a minimum of one day off in between for rest and recovery. So if you start with three days a week of a more intense workout, try to sneak in a 20 minute walk on two other days. It doesn't have to be as strenuous as your other workouts, but definitely try to do something for 20-30 minutes to get your body moving and your heart rate up.

Overall, it depends on your goals. If you're just going for general overall health, five days of light to moderate exercise for 30 minutes per day will do it. However, if you are looking to really improve overall fitness and really tone up your problem areas, you need to do at least five days at a higher intensity lasting from 30-60 minutes.

If you’re already doing five days at a higher intensity, don’t worry. These workouts I’ve created will help you change it up without adding extra time to your already jammed schedule.

Just know that at the end of the day, unless you’re a professional athlete or training for a distance race, there really is no benefit in working out more than five days a week - or for longer than 60 minutes in a single workout. Seriously.

Regardless of how many days you workout, I think you should be proud of yourself for doing it! It's not easy to make the commitment to yourself and get out there. So whatever you do, be proud of yourself!

ESTABLISHING A ROUTINE

Whether you're just getting started working out, eating right, or just adding some new moves to your repertoire, you need to figure out how to build this new habit into your already established routine.

After all, old habits are hard to break, and adding new ones isn't easy either. So the real question is: how long do you have to be consistent before it stops taking a ton of self-control, will power, and commitment in order to stick to your plan?

Because just saying you're going to do it isn't enough.

In fact, if you do a quick Google search, you'll see that it takes anywhere from 21 to 28 days to establish a new habit.

Personally, I don't think 21 days is enough.

I've seen grown women absolutely stressed out beyond belief at the idea of giving up their daily caffeine fix or laying off the junk food. And once they decide to do it, it takes them longer than 21 days to adjust, detox and change their mindset.

It's more about how dedicated you are about pursuing and reaching your goal.

According to research conducted by Phillippa Lally and colleagues from University College London (Lally et al. 2009) it takes 66 days or roughly two months to establish a new habit or routine.

That means you need to make a commitment to your new workout and eating habits for at least 2 months for them to really take hold. I've even seen cases in which it may take up to 90 days. So doing something new for a few days, or even a week or two, or three, won't be enough for it to become a habit.

So take an honest look at your schedule and figure out where you can fit your workouts in and earmark those times for working out. If you're working on improving your diet, like increasing your water intake or adding in more leafy greens, figure out how and where you can make those changes. Then make yourself a chart and check off when you've either completed a workout or did something good for your diet.

This way, you can start tracking your progress and it will also help keep you focused on your goal.

The simple act of writing something down and then checking it off once completed is known to increase your sense of satisfaction and acts as good reinforcement too!

JUST GET OUT THERE & DO IT!

So now you know your goals and what you want to accomplish. You've set your schedule and figured out how to fit your workouts in. You've identified where you need to make changes to your diet. Now, you've got to actually get out there and do it.

If you're trying something new, whether it's hitting the gym for the first time in years or eating a salad for lunch when you've had a burger every day for years, there's always a feeling of self-consciousness.

Let me tell you, that's perfectly normal.

Now, let me tell you something else. Get over it.

No one is staring at your butt and talking about how huge it is. Or laughing at what you look like as you run. Or wondering what someone like you is doing working out or eating a salad. You're not too fat, too slow, too uncoordinated or whatever it is that you think you are.

Plus, they've all got their own issues.

Let me tell you my own story. Growing up, I was taught that I should try to be perfect at everything. I was also taught to avoid anything that would draw attention to myself. Talk about a recipe for poor self-esteem. Let's just say confidence wasn't my thing. It's very hard for me to try new things, particularly when people can watch and have the opportunity to "judge." I grew up to be very self-conscious and always thought people were watching everything that I did.

I tried a few times in high school and college to work out. I was on the track team and tried running a few times, but never stuck with it. I wasn't very good and I felt like everyone was laughing and making fun of how bad I was.

Plus, I didn't really care for sweat.

After college, I started working at a desk job and got it into my head that I was going to work out. I'm not sure why. I just felt like it was something I should do. Maybe it was because I was feeling my butt start to spread from too much time in front of a computer.

So I decided to join an all-female gym. It seemed less intimidating somehow. The first day I went there I was so nervous; I thought everyone would know I was new. What a crazy thought! Of course they thought I was new! They never saw me before. I stood in the back and did my best to follow along in step class, bumbling, stumbling and tripping my way through.

And you know what? No one laughed. No one pointed or snickered or even gave me a sideways glance. No one cared that I couldn't get all the moves.

So I came back the next day. And then the next. Now 20 plus years later, I'm a fitness instructor myself. Who knew?

Here's something I figured out: you want to know why no one laughed? In fact, why no one even paid me any attention? They were too worried about themselves and people looking at THEM to bother paying any attention to ME.

Not convinced? Well, here's another story for you. When I was a grad school student in my early 30s, I decided I wanted to run in a real race. Even though I'd been working out for years, and was in decent shape, I didn't have the confidence to go outside and run. I mean to jog on a treadmill in a gym is one thing, but to do it out in public, *where everyone can see you*, is another. I mean, any running event always has bystanders who watch. I was really self-conscious. All of my old insecurities came back and I just couldn't do it.

What if I couldn't finish it? What if I had to walk? What if I came in last? What if people laughed? I had myself convinced that people would laugh and point at me if I ever dared to run outside in public. Plus, why did I even think I would be able to run that far? How dare I think that I could do this? Running is for other, fitter people. Not me.

So I put the idea of race on a back burner.

Luckily however, over the course of getting my degree, I became friends with a woman who was training for her second marathon. Not just any marathon either: The Chicago marathon. She was such a normal girl. Not particularly thin. You wouldn't look at her and instantly think she's a runner. For some reason, the thought that a normal girl like her could do it inspired me and gave me confidence. I made a split-second decision and decided I was going to do it too. I signed up for the Chicago marathon before I could change my mind.

Whatever possessed me to sign up for a marathon when I had never run more than 2 miles, let alone any type of race, even a one mile fun run, I don't know. I just knew that I wanted to do it. Or at least try.

By the way, if you don't know the length of a marathon, it's 26.2 miles. Trust me, it's a long way to run.

I could bore you with my many training stories here, but I'll save that for another day. Let's just suffice it to say I trained and got ready for the race.

Come race day, I had absolutely no idea what I was in for. I was as nervous as all get out. I mean I was going to attempt to run 26.2 miles in front of an expected crowd of close to one million spectators. That is no place for a girl who doesn't like to do things in public that she isn't perfect at or doesn't do very well. Not to mention I had never run a race before in my life. I kept thinking, "I'm not a runner. What the %$#!*& did I get myself into????"

The thought, "I don't know if I can do this" kept rolling through my head. I was full of self-doubt even though I had trained for months.

Well, someone must have noticed how nervous I was and asked if this was my first time. When I responded yes, I got the surprise of my life. Not only did that person give me encouragement, so did all the other people around me who heard it was my first time. They even told me about their first times. Turns out, they all felt the same exact way I did right then.

Even the crowds were amazing. They cheered for all of us as we went by. When I ran, they cheered. When I walked, they cheered. Everyone, from fellow racers to bystanders, just encouraged me and told me I could do it. No one laughed at me. Not once. No one cared that I wasn't the skinniest or very fast. They all just honestly were cheering for me. For ***all*** of us who ran.

I no longer do many races, as I have some hip and heart issues that prevent me from doing them. But I still love to cheer people on! Whether you're first, last or in the middle I remember how much it helped and I'm happy to see other people get out there. I want to pass on the same good wishes that were given to me all those years ago.

Now, you may not want to run a marathon. Or maybe you do. That's not the point. I'm telling you this story because it has a great lesson that I think is important for you to know. You see, anyone who does any kind of event or sport remembers what it's like to be new. For the most part, racers of any sport tend to be a friendly bunch. Plus, they know the more they encourage, the better you'll feel and the more races that you'll do. That's how the sport continues.

As for those bystanders? They're really there to cheer you on! They're not going to make fun of you. Why? Because you're doing something that they can't do. You're putting yourself out there. You're the one doing the race.

Why am I telling you all this? Because I know first-hand how you can self-sabotage yourself. I've done it to myself. And I've seen it repeatedly with the women I've worked with.

Don't let your own insecurities stop you. So start lifting, running, riding, taking yoga or whatever it is you want to do. Just get out there and do it. No, you won't be perfect the first time (or second or even the third time you do it). But you'll get better each time. Remember, we all have to start somewhere.

NUTRITION 101

First, let me say, if you're looking for a totally done-for-you diet plan, telling you exactly how, what, when and where to eat for the next 30 days, then this isn't the book for you.

Why is that? Because I believe that if I tell you exactly what to put in your mouth, you'll never really learn how to make decisions on your own. I can't be with you at every restaurant, party, book club, or BBQ. Plus, I can't possibly list every type of food you'll ever come across.

In other words, you need to do learn to take your diet into your own hands.

Not to mention, we all have different preferences and tastes. You may be a meat eater or maybe you're a vegetarian. Or maybe there are just certain foods you just don't like. For me, I personally hate beans: kidney, lima, pinto and even tofu. I absolutely hate them. I don't like them, never have, never will.

Although for some reason, green beans are OK.

I know that beans are a good source of fiber and protein. They're a healthy part of a balanced diet. But I do not care that they are good for me. I absolutely, positively cannot stand them. I don't care about their numerous health benefits or how nutritious they are. There is no way you're going to make me eat them.

You probably have things you hate too. Not to mention, some of us are lactose or gluten intolerant, or have a whatever intolerance. I can't possibly prescribe a one size fits all diet here. It would never work.

Rather, I want to give you guidelines and really educate you about nutrition. That way, you can make informed decisions based on your own personal likes and dislikes.

Now, there are all kinds of experts touting all kinds of ways to eat. There's vegan, vegetarian, juicing, and Paleo. There are also more weight management companies than I can even count.

I think there are pros and cons to all of these different types of “diets” or ways of eating. It’s not for me to tell you that vegan (where you eat no animal products of any kind) is better than eating Paleo (a diet based on what the cavemen ate), or being a carnivore is the way to go instead of becoming a vegetarian. That’s a matter of personal choice.

However, no matter what you eat, I DO believe you should be eating clean.

Clean eating simply means eating food in its most natural state. In other words, it means avoiding processed foods.

I truly believe that eliminating processed foods from your diet is the #1 thing that you can to improve your overall health. Even if this is the only thing you do, you will see a tremendous difference in how you feel. I couldn’t believe the difference in my own body when I did it years ago.

I just felt so much better; I didn’t feel so weighed down. I had more energy. Overall, I just felt lighter and healthier, not to mention, my stomach pudge decreased. An extra bonus!

What does processed really mean? It's more than just fast food, Oreos, potato chips, and soda (all things to avoid, or at least to not eat very much of, by the way!).

Some consider processed foods to be those that have added preservatives or are made from ingredients that have long shelf lives. While that's certainly true, there's more to it than that.

The true meaning of processed is a food that has been altered in any way from its true original form. In other words, if it doesn't grow on a tree, bush, from the ground, or if it doesn't have a mother, then it's considered processed.

To me, there are various levels of "processed." For example, in the US, milk is pasteurized to kill bacteria, making it a processed food. Does that mean you should totally drop milk from your diet? Not necessarily. It's still a great form a dairy.

What about things like tofu? Eggs? Orange juice? How about a salad with grilled chicken from a fast food restaurant?

It really starts to get gray doesn't it? It's crazy!

Between all the different brands, packaging and claims, it's tough sometimes to know what's right and what's wrong; that's what is so freaking frustrating. You think you're doing something good, but it turns out you're really not.

Take a nutrition bar. Now, there are a lot of great bars out there. The brands Lara and Kind put out great bars that have healthy, natural ingredients that are pretty close to their natural form. But then there are bars by Cliff and Kellogg that I avoid. Why? Because even though they contain many good ingredients, they also contain a whole lot of artificial ones along with preservatives.

That's why you've really got to take matters into your own hands. Luckily, I've learned an easy way to demystify the whole process when you're in the grocery store. Simply read the list of ingredients. If you don't can't pronounce and/or understand all of the ingredients, put it back. It's probably got something in it you shouldn't put in your body.

If you're currently eating clean, good for you. If you're not, don't feel like you need to jump on the band wagon all at once. It's a process. The point is to get started. Take baby steps and start moving forward. Start by eliminating one type of processed food and let your body adjust. Then eliminate another, and so on and so on until you finally eliminate most, if not all, from your diet.

This isn't a contest, simply move at your own speed to do what works best for you.

Your body and your health will thank you.

DIET PROGRAMS

I'm going to keep this portion short, because I've already covered a lot in the previous chapter. But if you're at a place with your nutrition where you really feel like you need some additional assistance, then read on.

Maybe you know you suck at portion control. Or you know that you honestly just need someone to tell you exactly what to eat and when. Well then, you may just want to try a diet program.

If you can, I always recommend working with a certified nutritionist. They are professionals that are specifically trained to work with you to create a balanced diet that works for you. They can help get to the root of some of the reasons your diet is suffering and come up with a program that you can stick with.

However, maybe you don't want to work one on one with a nutritionist because of the time, money or maybe you just don't want to do it for whatever reason. In that case, I highly recommend Weight Watchers.

Why Weight Watchers? The reason I like Weight Watchers is because they have created programs that teach you how to eat. They don't give you prepackaged meal plans. You learn portion control, how to work in the treats as well as the types of food you should eat based on the foods you like. However, you will still keep in mind my advice for eating clean.

My final piece of advice? Stop looking at this as a diet. I know that you've probably heard this before, but it's so true. When you think of the word diet, you automatically think of deprivation. Also, you tend to think that it's short term. It's not. Instead, what you really need to do is learn a new way of eating; one that can work for you the rest of your life. And that's the real reason I recommend a nutritionist or Weight Watchers. I think they're the best for helping you learn how to eat in a way that will help you reach your goals not only now, but also help you keep them in the long run.

THE HOT SPOTS

I'm not talking about your belly or thighs here! I'm talking about the things you do to sabotage your diet.

Over the years, I've gotten many questions about food and eating right. That's why I want to address some of the big reasons women get themselves into trouble without even trying. Now, some of these things aren't backed up by science, and all of these are certainly my opinions to be sure. But I've been in and around the fitness field for 20 years and these are what I've found to be some of the biggest ways women sabotage themselves.

- ***Skipping meals.*** Yes, we're all guilty of skipping a meal here and there. Life gets busy, right? The problem is, if you skip a meal, you typically just end up hungrier later. When later happens, and when we finally do eat, we either eat more than we should to compensate or because we're so flipping hungry, we just stuff our faces with anything and everything. At this point, we really don't care what we put in our mouths so of course we tend to just eat the wrong thing in general. Which all means more calories (and probably more fat, sugar and salt too). So eat breakfast. And lunch. And yes, dinner too. I'm not even going to go into why breakfast is the most important meal of the day...
- ***Cutting calories too far.*** We all know that we need to consume fewer calories and move our bodies more to lose weight. So it stands to reason that the more you cut, the

more you'll lose, right? Wrong! While that will happen at first, if you keep up those low calorie counts, it will eventually stall over time. This typically happens when individuals try to consume less than 1,000 calories a day. That's because when you get to this low of a calorie count, your body goes into starvation mode. In starvation mode, your body starts hoarding calories, and shuts down the metabolism. The end result? A scale that doesn't budge no matter how little you eat or how much you work out. So if you're looking to lose weight over the long term, shoot for 1,500 calories a day. If you really want to go lower, try not to go below 1,200 calories, unless you have a medical reason, of course.

- ***Drinking calories.*** I'm talking about drinks with calories. Like a big glass of juice or a Starbucks coffee drink. A 16 ounce glass of juice can have over 250 calories and the same size Starbucks can have several hundred calories. Why waste your calories on a drink? It's not going to fill you up. Plus, it's so much more satisfying to chew on food than it is to drink something. I'm not talking low calorie treats, like a diet mocha or something with 150-200 calories. That's fine from time to time (not every day of course!). You need to watch those sugary and alcoholic drinks. They can cause the calories to creep up. Best choice? Stick with water.

- ***Denial***. Da'Nile is more than a river in Egypt. It's also alive and well right in your home. Yes, there are calories in condiments. No, not all salads are healthy…especially when they have French fries, bacon, and cheese and are topped off with a creamy dressing. And yes, food that you eat with friends or those quick tastes you snatch as you cook dinner definitely have calories. No matter what you tell yourself, just know everything that you put in your mouth, EVERYTHING, counts. Sad, but true...
- ***Not reading labels.*** Seriously. You not only need to read them but you also need to learn to understand them so you know what you're putting in your mouth. I know it's hard, but it does get easier. Even if you check nothing else on a label, at least check the calories per serving size and the amount of servings per packet. A serving may have 200 calories, but if you eat the whole bag, and the bag is worth 5 servings, you just wrecked your diet no matter how healthy something is.

LABELS DEMYSTIFIED

That last point leads me right into this topic: Labels. If you're like me, you try to eat healthy. Or at least you know you should. It's just that sometimes it's so hard! Plus, the labels don't always seem to help. Free, Low, Lean, Light... the list goes on and on.

What do all of those food terms on labels really mean? Trust me when I say that they don't all mean "healthy." The best way to be healthy is to be armed with the right information. So let's go through a brief explanation of some of the terms you should be familiar with.

Before we can get started on terms, let's break down the actual nutrition label. Now, I know most of you know how to read a label. But a refresher never hurts!

I like to think of food labels as a table of contents such as you'd see in a book. The job of the label is to tell you exactly what is inside.

Now, the information provided is based on a 2,000 calorie food intake for a typical adult. The daily value gives you an idea of a food's nutrient contribution to your diet; 5% or less is considered low for that nutrient, 10% to 19% is good, and 20% or more is high.

Over 40 Fact - On average, a woman consumes about 2,000 calories a day just to maintain her current weight. So if you're trying to lose a few pounds, adjust accordingly!

Most nutrients are measured in **grams**, also written as **g** or **gr**. Some nutrients are measured in **milligrams**, or **mg**. Just like the name suggests, milligrams are smaller than grams. In fact, they're very tiny. There are 1,000 milligrams in 1 gram. And you thought you didn't understand the metric system, right?

Other information such as fat, protein, carbohydrates, and sodium are given in **percentages**, which helps you see how they stack up against your recommended daily intake.

Finally, underneath the label, you'll typically see the ingredient list. Ingredients are listed in order of decreasing weight in the product. I always make sure to scan this as well, just because I like to check the quality of the ingredients. Personally, I like to know exactly what I'm putting in my body. Don't forget my earlier explanation regarding the importance of being able to pronounce and understand all the ingredients. But I leave that choice up to you!

FREE - Here's the one that has the potential to be the most confusing. I don't know about you, but when I see the word free, I think FREE! In other words, I would think the word free = zero.

That's almost true, but not quite.

Essentially when you see the word free in a label or description it means that the product doesn't contain any amount of, or only a trace amount of, one of the following compounds: fat, saturated fat, cholesterol, sodium, sugars and calories. To make matters worse, you may also see free foods labeled "without," "no" and "zero" which can also means "free." Just know that the word “free” doesn’t mean 100%. For the most part, it’s close enough, though.

Here are some examples:

- ***Calorie-Free*** - fewer than 5 calories per serving
- ***Sugar-Free*** - less than .5 grams per serving
- ***Fat-Free*** - less than .5 grams per serving

You’re probably thinking great, right? That’s because many foods labeled as “Free” represent a healthy choice and because of their lower fat, sugar and/or calories they can really help you lose those unwanted extra pounds. Just because they’re labeled “Free,” don’t think that these foods mean you get a dietary free for all. Just because it says free that doesn’t mean that it is an instant health food. There’s a dirty little secret too.

Want me to clue you in on what it is? The dirty little secret is that many food manufacturers tend to compensate for the loss of one thing by adding more of something else. Sugar-Free foods may have added sodium. Fat-Free might have extra sugar or salt. So you really have to read your labels and watch out. You might want to lose weight, but those extras can wreak havoc on your body too. Another unfortunate thing about Free foods? It's that Free foods can also mean “taste free.” Fat free cheese anyone?

LOW - The next step up (or down depending on how you look at it) from “Free” is “Low.” Makes sense, right? “Low” is the term typically used to describe foods that can be eaten frequently without exceeding dietary guidelines for one or more of these components: fat, saturated fat, cholesterol, sodium and/or calories. Again, just like the term “Free” has multiple synonyms, the term “Low” can be interchangeable with words such as "little," "few" and "low source of."

- ***Low fat*** - 3 grams or less per serving
- ***Low saturated fat*** - 1 gram or less per serving
- ***Low sodium*** - 140 milligrams or less per serving
- ***Very low sodium*** - 35 milligrams or less per serving
- ***Low cholesterol*** - 20 milligrams or less and 2 grams or less of saturated fat per serving
- ***Low calorie*** - 40 calories or less per serving

I think most foods that have this label tend to taste better than their "free" counterparts. When they're used in a recipe, you often can't even tell. They're a great way to lower your daily caloric intake. However, you still need to be on the lookout to make sure a manufacturer hasn't compensated by adding something you don't want, such as extra sugar or salt.

Over 40 NOTE: Other than the dairy case, typically when you see the word Free or Low used in the label it's a manufactured food product. I'm a big fan of eating food as close to the original form as possible. So shop in the fresh food area as much as possible.

LEAN - You typically don't see this term regarding fresh fruits, vegetables, dairy or grains. Instead, this term generally refers to the amount (or lack thereof) of fat in meat, fish and seafood.

The two most common terms you'll see are:

- ***Lean*** - less than 10 grams of fat, 4.5 or less of saturated fat and less than 95 milligrams of cholesterol per serving and per 100 grams; and
- ***Extra Lean*** - less than 5 grams of fat, less than 2 grams of saturated fat and less than 95 milligrams cholesterol per serving and per 100 grams.

To have a lean body, it makes sense that you want to eat lean too, right? That's why you want to try to put lean animal proteins into your body. There have been multiple studies done showing that leaner cuts of meat are better for your health in more ways than one. However, while that logic applies to land animals, it doesn't necessarily apply to fish.

For example, salmon is a fish with higher fat content, but it's high in healthy fats. Meat, especially red meat, doesn't work like that. So if you're used to eating fattier cuts, such as rib-eye or skirt steaks, try filets instead. Go for 90% or higher in your ground meats. Also, when eating ground turkey or chicken, make sure to get the white breast meat. Yes, it will cost more and it may take your taste buds a little adjusting, but it's better for your health and will help keep calories down.

There are many other terms out there, but here are some of the most common. I've listed them in a somewhat descending order:

High - This term can be used if the food contains 20 percent or more of the daily value for a particular nutrient in a serving. This is a great label if you're looking to add more of a particular nutrient into your diet.

Good Source - This is the next step down from "High." The term "Good Source" means that one serving contains 10-19 percent of the Daily Value for a particular nutrient. For example, cereal boxes may say "good source of fiber."

Reduced - This term means that a nutritionally altered product contains at least 25 percent less of a nutrient or calories as compared to the regular or reference product. However, a reduced claim can't be made for a product if its reference food already meets the requirement for a low claim.

Less/Lower - These two terms are interchangeable. This means that a food, whether altered or not, contains 25 percent less of a nutrient or calories as compared to the reference food; For example, pretzels that have 25 percent less fat than potato chips. "Fewer" is another acceptable synonym for less.

Light - This word can mean two things. A nutritionally altered product contains one-third fewer calories or one-half the fat of the reference food. If the food derives 50 percent or more of the calories from fat, the reduction must be 50 percent of the fat.

Second, the sodium content of a low-calorie, low-fat food has been reduced by 50 percent. The term "light" can still be used to describe properties such as texture and color as long as the label explains the intent. For example: 'light brown sugar.'

Percent Fat-Free - A product that uses this term must be a low-fat or fat-free product. The claim must accurately represent the amount of fat present in 100 grams of the food. So, if the box of cookies you are picking up says 95 percent fat-free, it must contain 5 grams of fat per 100 grams.

WHAT TO PUT IN YOUR MOUTH

Now that you know the terms and some of the things we all tend to do to sabotage our diets, it's time to learn what it is we really should be putting in our mouth and eating.

Now, I readily admit that I'm not a registered dietician or nutritionist. In fact, I encourage you to go visit one if you're really in need of some personalized help and direction on this topic. Especially if you have a medical condition, question or concern.

Over the years, I've learned quite a few things about healthy eating along with what works and what doesn't. So, while I'm not going to give a prescribed way of eating, I am going to share with you my top nine tips for eating healthy and staying on track.

Tip #1 - You Need to Consume Calories.
Now, in the previous chapter I talked a lot about eating and calories. Please, PLEASE

make sure that you are eating at least 1200 calories a day, unless of course, you are under the care and supervision of a physician. Ideally you should be consuming between 1200 and 1500 for weight loss depending on your size. But I know that there are a few of you who are going too low on your calorie count, thinking that it will get you to your goal that much quicker.

However, believe me when I say that there is a law of diminishing return.

Just like too many calories can cause you to gain, not enough can sabotage your diet just as easily. Without enough calories coming in, your body goes in to starvation mode. When it does that, your metabolism shuts down because the body starts to hold on to anything and everything that you put into it. Why? Because your body is super smart and it picks up fast that it's not getting all that much food so it seeks to conserve. And that's not what you are looking for.

So make sure that you are eating between 300 to 400 calories per meal plus a few snacks. 200 calories from one of those freezer meals does not a meal make; that's a snack. So make sure that you are eating enough.

Here's a few ways to bump it up and get some more energy: Look for protein like cheese, yogurt, and even nuts. Just make sure you watch the portions; it's a quick and healthy way to add some calories in a manner that's good for you too.

Tip #2 - You really are what you eat. I'm not just talking calories; I'm talking quality. So are you still eating processed foods? Even just a teeny, tiny bit? Diet coke maybe? A 100 calorie snack pack to get you over the hump? If you are, please stop! These processed foods and chemicals are sabotaging your diet and your waistline. You need to eat clean.

Let me explain. I'm a big believer in dropping processed foods. Why? I want you to look the world over at all the different ways people survive and even thrive. There's an area in Switzerland where they eat primarily raw milk and cream; then there's the high fat, high protein of the Inuit; the high animal protein of the Massai of Kenya and Tanzania; as well as the high carb, low fat of South Africans.

The diets may vary greatly, but they do all have one thing in common. Can you guess what it is?

They are all natural diets. No sugars (especially the refined white stuff) and no processed foods.

The result? These people don't suffer nearly as much as Americans from high blood pressure, cancer, cardiovascular disease, diabetes, osteoporosis or obesity. And if they have access to good medical care, their longevity is very similar to ours - except they are a whole lot healthier.

Why? They are eating pure, unprocessed foods.

It makes sense. Eating pure, real, unprocessed foods is almost always the best thing for your body, no matter what style of diet you choose to follow.

Now some of these cultures don't have much of a choice in how they eat. They are extremely dependent on their environment. But luckily, we have access to a wide variety of foods. There's the good and the bad. You really have to choose. It's up to you.

I am going to borrow a quote from Jack LaLanne here. He's considered the godfather of fitness for those of you who don't know him. When he died at the ripe old age of 96, he still looked amazing, and had a body that many a 30 year old could only wish for; Google or Bing him to find out more. He's quite an inspiration. But he says, and I quote, "If God made it, good. If man made it, bad." There's a lot of truth in that statement. I use it all the time myself when I'm food shopping. It's easy and basic enough to understand, even when you feel overwhelmed by choices. So if you go by that, you can't go wrong.

Trust me, you'll feel and look a lot better.

Tip #3 - Shop the perimeter of the store. It's the easiest way I've found to avoid the processed foods. The perimeter of the store tends to be where they keep things with a shorter shelf life such as fresh fruits and vegetables, dairy, lean proteins, and freshly baked grains. The interior aisles hold all things that are considered “shelf stable.” In other words, many things there contain ingredients that make them last longer.

So if you stay on the outside aisles of the store you’ll get yourself into a whole lot less trouble!

Tip #4 - Carbs are the NOT the devil! One of the things that I hear repeatedly from women is how they dropped all carbs. While I’m not going to argue with you about dropping the white bread, I AM going to tell you that not all carbs are created equal. In fact, your body needs them to function properly.

There are actually two types of carbs, simple and complex. Neither is bad.

Simple carbs get a bad rap, and that's because most of us think of them as processed foods, such as white bread, baked goods, jams and table sugars. But even in this category, there are good simple carbs too (which basically means fruit). They are low in simple sugars, have loads of fiber, vitamins and minerals and are easily broken down and utilized by the body. In other words, they're good for you!

Then there are complex carbs. Complex means that it takes your body longer to break them down, giving you a steady stream of energy throughout the day. Natural, unprocessed carbs are devoid of artificial colorings and preservatives as well. Think of foods like brown rice, brans, muesli, baked potato with skin, lentils, root vegetables (with skin), beans, and non-instant oatmeal.

According to the food pyramid, you're shooting for 6-11 servings PER DAY combined of simple (the good kind) and complex carbs. So one or two slices of wheat bread during the day along some oatmeal for breakfast won't cut it; you've got to incorporate it into each meal. Do a meal with grilled chicken or fish, brown rice and green beans to grab a quick two servings. Snack on fruit at least 2x per day.

Both the complex and good simple carbs contain vitamins, minerals, phytochemicals and other nutrients that are rarely present in simple-sugar food items. They help keep your energy more stable as well and can really fill you up.

As a fellow fruit lover, just be forewarned: although fruits are considered good simple carbs, and are a great choice, don't lean on them too heavily. Fruit typically contains lots of natural sugars (which is probably why I like them!). Unfortunately, just like the bad simple carbs, these sugars too can turn into fat if you have too many. So try to stick to the 2-4 serving a day recommended by the FDA.

Tip #5 - Follow the 80/20 Rule. I'm a big believer in the 80/20. I'm a realist after all. I'm human and so are you. Just like you, I have a soft spot for some foods I know I shouldn't eat. I know I'm not going to eat correctly 100% of the time ALL the time; it's just not gonna happen. Most of us aren't. Let's face it, if you deprive yourself of the stuff you really want all the time, when you finally do allow yourself to have it, you're probably going to go overboard. And that is its own slippery slope. Plus, that's no way to live.

That's why I recommend the 80/20 rule. Strive to eat right 80% of the time: Lean protein, complex carbs and plenty of fruits and veggies. The other 20% of the time, give yourself the treats. It makes it so much easier to stay on track if you allow yourself some treats from time to time.

To me, my 20% includes wine and chocolate. Not to mention an occasional forage into a bag of Doritos too if I'm being honest. To you, that might mean something totally different. It doesn't matter; we all have foods that we love that we know we shouldn't eat. The point is to allow yourself to have them from time to time so you recognize that they are a treat.

I always recommend eating right Monday through Friday then allowing yourself the treats on the weekend. Weekends are typically a time to let loose and socialize, so it's the easiest and best to time to loosen up the rules! If you ate properly throughout the work week, you'll be able to indulge with friends and family without guilt. Just remember that this isn't a free license to totally let loose. You still need to look at these times as treats.

Tip #6 - Learn to count & read. Yes, I know you can read. You're reading this book after all! And yes, I know that you can count too. But now, what I really want, is for you to read labels and count your food. It really makes a difference.

Check your labels. Let's say you're a chip lover and that is where you're going to allow yourself some treats. The label says that a serving of your favorite chips equals 14 chips and 160 calories. Now reach into the bag, count and pull 14 chips out. That's your serving.

This goes for everything.

Now, I'm not saying get a scale and measure positively everything. Although if you know that you have trouble gaging your portions, then be sure to invest in one. It may be just the thing you need to keep your diet in check. However, what I'm really saying is to be aware of a serving size so you understand where your calories are coming from.

I know that this is a lot to digest (no pun intended!). That's why I've included a weekly food log at the end of this chapter as well as at the end of this book for you to use. I know it can seem cumbersome and be a bit of a pain. But doing it for just a week can be a big eye opener as to how you're really eating and where you're falling short.

Tip #7 - Drink Your Water. One of the best things that you can for yourself is to drink water. It's good for your whole body and flushes out all the nasty toxins we ingest either through diet or our environment. It also helps with muscle fatigue and soreness by helping to lube the joints and muscles, keeping them fluid and pliable instead of tight and stiff.

Not enough to persuade you to drink up? Water also helps to burn fat and build muscle. If this isn't your incentive, I don't know what is. ***This means drinking water will help you lose weight!!!!*** Who knew there was magic in your very own home?

Now, when I say water, I mean actual water, not just any liquid. Your water intake does not include your cup of coffee or tea nor your soda or juice. Yes, those are liquids. But count those separate. I'm talking WATER!

There are those of you who are good girls and drink your water daily. But there are those, maybe you, who know drinking water is good for you, but don't do it.

Really, you can't get much easier and cheaper than water. It's right in your own sink. If you don't like the taste, add lemon or lime to it for a bit of punch. And if you have a few hundred dollars to spare, get a water system put in. Where I live in California, our public water has so many things added to it that it truly tastes terrible. Even my dogs won't drink it. I installed a water system in my home for about $200 and it really makes the water taste fantastic.

But at the end of the day, just suck it up and drink it. You're a grown up girl. You know sometimes you just have to do things that you don't like because they are good for you. And honestly, the more you drink it, the more you will like it. So drink up!!!

What's the right amount? I'm sure you've heard 64 ounces, or even just drinking it when you're thirsty. However, it's easy to confuse thirst with hunger. So if you are feeling a bit hungry, try boosting the water intake and see if it helps; it just might do the trick.

So to make sure you're getting enough I always recommend dividing your weight by 2 and that's the number of ounces you should shoot for. So if you weigh 140 pounds, you should consume at least 70 ounces a day.

Tip #8 - Go for Color. Turns out, the more color food has, the more nutrients it contains. So look at your plate. Is it colorful? Or is there a little too much beige? Not that beige is bad. There are some great foods that are a little lacking in color. Think dairy, eggs, and potatoes (skin on please). For the most part, beige foods tend to be stripped of some, if not all, of their essential vitamins and nutrients. The wider the variety of colors that you include in your meal, the more likely you're getting all of the nutrients you need. Not to mention that it's a lot more pleasing to the eye!

Tip #9 - Eat Your Fruits and Veggies. I've looked at many food logs in my day, and one thing I've noticed is that we as women aren't eating all of our fruits and veggies. If you're already eating your five, good for you! If not, it's time to add them in. Here's the great thing about this:

You should shoot for two to three servings of fruit and three or more servings of veggies. It's not as hard as it sounds. For the most part, a fruit and/or veggie serving is about one half of a cup. Add a slice of lettuce and tomato to your sandwich and presto! How about a big salad? Depending on the size, it's probably at least 2-3 servings.

Over 40 Note - Hate to eat plain fruits and veggies? Try a smoothie! It's a great way to sneak them in.

Here's my quick way to get most of my servings in using just one simple drink; it's my very own green smoothie recipe:

Debby's Sneaky Smoothie

In a blender add:

1 banana
1 cup strawberries

1/2-1 cup raspberries
1-2 cups spinach
1 cup almond milk
Blend until smooth

It's a smooth and creamy drink that's good for you and tastes like a treat. It's got 3 servings of fruit and up to two servings of veggies. Drink this and you only need one more serving of veggies for the day!

Don't let the spinach scare you. When you add berries, especially tart ones like raspberries, you really can't taste it! Just make sure to add less spinach to start and work your way up. If you don't like raspberries, you can always try lime or lemon juice instead to balance out the bitterness of the greens, or really any fruit that has a tartness to it.

Not to mention, it's super easy with minimal clean up. Just throw everything in your blender and turn it on. I even add the green tops of the berries for extra greens. Plus, you can use fresh or frozen berries, although if you use frozen, make sure to add some extra water too as it gets a little thick. You can also change it up with any type of fruit that you like (although

I always recommend a banana as it gives it a truly creamy, almost milkshake like taste. Not to mention the potassium is good for those working muscles!).

You'll see that I don't add things like protein powder and the like. That goes back to my philosophy on processed foods. I consider most protein powder to be processed, as it is far from its natural state, so I don't typically use it. However, when I know I've been working out extra hard and need the extra protein I will add some of Nutiva's Organic Hemp Shake in Vanilla, which also comes in chocolate and berry. But I find the vanilla to change the flavor of my smoothie the least. If you'd like to try a protein powder, this is the one that I really recommend.

I also personally use almond milk. You could also use soy (just don't use the flavored as it has lots of extra sugar) or any other low-fat or fat-free milk. But all of this is truly a personal decision.

Now, I know that you may be tempted to use juice for the liquid instead of almond, soy, or dairy milk. Don't. It won't be as creamy, plus it adds more sugar that this smoothie really doesn't need. The fruit already gives it plenty.

Another recipe staple in my house is Tuscan Stew. This recipe is based off of one I found by Giada DeLaurentis. It's another way to get your veggies and it tastes absolutely fabulous. In fact, I've even made it for people of all ages, kids included, and everyone always loves it.

Tuscan Stew

1 rotisserie chicken OR 2-3 chicken breasts with skin (optional)
1-2 cans white beans, rinsed (optional)
1 small onion chopped
2 stalks celery chopped
4 carrots chopped
3-4 cloves garlic chopped
1 28 oz can chopped tomatoes
1 32 oz box of organic chicken broth
salt, pepper, basil

If using a rotisserie chicken, rough chop chicken into bite size pieces. Reserve the breast skin, keeping it as intact as possible. If using uncooked chicken breasts, cook for 20 minutes at 350 with drizzle of olive oil, salt and pepper. When cooled, remove skin and set aside to reserve. Rough chop the breasts into bite size pieces.

Chop onion, celery, and carrots to desired size; any size really works here. If you're not a fan of one of these vegetables, just chop it really fine. That way when it cooks, you won't really even notice it's there. I personally hate the taste and texture of celery, so I chop it extra fine and I can't even taste it.

Over 40 Note - A pre-made Mirapoix mix is a great time saver. Most grocery stores have it in the premade produce section. Mirapoix is chopped onion, celery and carrots. Just substitute those ingredients with one container.

Add 2 tbs. olive oil to pan and sauté vegetables until translucent, for about 10 minutes. Add chopped garlic and sauté for another 30 seconds. Add can of tomatoes and broth. Bring to a boil. Add the rinsed beans, chopped chicken and the skin you reserved.

Reduce heat to simmer and let cook for 25 minutes. Remove skin. Add salt, pepper, and basil (can use fresh or dry) to taste.

Again, here's the beauty of this one-pot meal: It's super easy if you use a rotisserie chicken or pre-cut veggies. You can also add any kind of veggies you want. Also, you can have chicken and beans or only chicken or only beans. Just make sure to add one of them for protein. It's the perfect one pot meal!

VITAMINS, HERBS, & SUPPLEMENTS OH MY!

Should you be taking a vitamin? Maybe. What about supplements? Perhaps. How about herbs? Depends.

Like how clearly I answer?

Probably not, but that's how I really feel.

To be honest, I don't have a problem with vitamins or supplements. I think they're a great way to get vital nutrients that you may not necessarily be getting from your diet.

You can find lots of debate on this topic on the Internet or even discussing it with doctors and/or scientists. Although most agree that they are beneficial, especially if you don't eat a healthy balanced diet. Since most people don't, or at least not every day, it's a simple and easy habit to get into to make sure that you're getting all the nutrients that your body needs.

That said, in speaking with my doctor, you should buy the best quality vitamin that you can; this isn't the time to always shop by price. I personally like Every Woman's One Daily by New Chapter. It's filled with lots of good stuff that you won't find in your typical vitamin, plus it's formulated for women over 40. They're also probiotic and made from organic fruits, vegetables and herbs.

Just be aware that there is truth to the statement that there can be too much of a good thing. Taking too much of any vitamin can actually be harmful. Just stay close to your recommend doses. So if you're taking a multivitamin or supplement, you don't need to eat cereal or drink juice that contains extra calcium or folic acid.

Forgotten Fundamentals

There are six fundamentals to fitness cardio, strength training, core, balance, flexibility, and of course, proper nutrition.

Out of those six, which ones do you think are most often overlooked, even among women who work out a regular basis?

They are balance and flexibility.

THE CASE FOR BALANCE

Balance is one of those things we all take for granted. In fact, I bet you probably don't think much about it. But balance is truly a critical piece of your body's overall fitness.

Why is balance so important? Because without balance, you'd fall over. In fact, every time you take a step forward, you're using balance to stay upright. Reaching over to grab something requires balance too.

Unfortunately, we all start losing our ability to balance as we age. Often, we don't even realize that it's gone before it's too late. That's why you often hear of healthy older people falling and breaking their hip; it's all due to balance. Luckily, it doesn't take much work to get it back.

So here's a quick way to work on improving your balance, no matter where you are on the spectrum. Just note that you may want to have something close by such as a table, chair, wall or pole that you can reach out and touch, especially if you are just starting to work on it.

Stand on a flat surface with both feet firmly planted on the ground. Then lift one foot off the ground. Keep that foot lifted for 20 seconds. Don't worry if you can't do it the first time; just touch your toes down as needed and then lift back up. Then reverse to the other foot.

Need more of a challenge? Then lift your foot or even your leg higher or try holding for up to a minute. Even better: Hold it as high as you can for one whole minute.

Once you're able to hold your leg up high for a whole minute, you can add on. Try continually lifting each leg for one minute. Or make small circles in the air with your toe.

Need more? Add it all together! Hold it for one minute, then do leg lifts for one minute, then do the small circles (each direction for one minute). That's a total of 4 minutes of balance on just one leg!

You'll be amazed by how quickly you'll improve your balance just by lifting your leg and holding it in place for 20 seconds.

FLEXIBILITY

The other crucial piece that is often forgotten is stretching. I don't understand why, especially when it feels so good!

But I get it. It takes time. And let's face it; we're all pressed for time. Or we're just simply too tired at the end of our workouts. However, stretching can help make sure our muscles stay pliable and flexible.

There's more to it than that; being flexible helps improve the muscle balance around a joint, which helps with posture. It also helps reduce the risk of injury when playing a sport, working out, or just doing regular chores around the house. It also helps to increase the blood and nutrient supply to muscles and cartilage, which helps reduce any muscle soreness after training.

But don't think that because you stretch you can't get injured. Stretching, for instance, won't prevent an overuse injury. Talk to your doctor or physical therapist about the best way to stretch if you have any health concerns.

There are lots of stretches, which I'll go over in more detail in the workout portion, but here are the five most important tips to remember about stretching.

Tip #1 - Never stretch cold. Meaning, don't jump right into stretching without warming up and getting the blood flowing first. A cold muscle is typically a tight muscle. Think about your muscle like a piece of chewing gum. Can you stretch a piece of gum when you first pull it out of the wrapper? No. It just breaks off. But once you begin to chew, it softens and become pliable. Your muscle is the same way; it needs to be warm to be pliable. Trying to stretch a cold muscle could lead to injury.

Tip #2 - Hold the stretch for 20-30 seconds. Why? Because you want to allow the muscle enough time to fully relax. Any less and again, the muscle will become more prone to injury. It could tighten further, or worse, it could snap and tear. Holding a stretch for 20-30 seconds helps make sure the stretch is effective.

Tip #3 - Never, ever press on a joint to stretch a muscle. You risk injury to the joint. Press on the actual muscle.

Tip #4 - Stretch to the point of tension, not pain. If a stretch hurts, back off. A stretch may be uncomfortable, but it should never, ever cause you pain.

Tip #5 - Stretch both sides equally. I know that this may sound silly, but don't forget to stretch both sides of your body. For example, if you stretch your right quadriceps, you should also stretch your left quadriceps. Even if you only feel tight on one side, stretch both. Trust me, both sides need it.

Want a simple stretch that works on almost your whole body? Try the total body stretch. Simply reach up to the sky while you lift up on your toes, raising your heels. (Shh, it's good for balance too). Then, bend over at the waist and try to touch your toes or your shins. Try not to bounce, just hold it nice and steady for 10-15 seconds at a time. Repeat at least twice per stretch so you get the full 20 to 30 seconds the muscles really need.

Example of Total Body Stretch

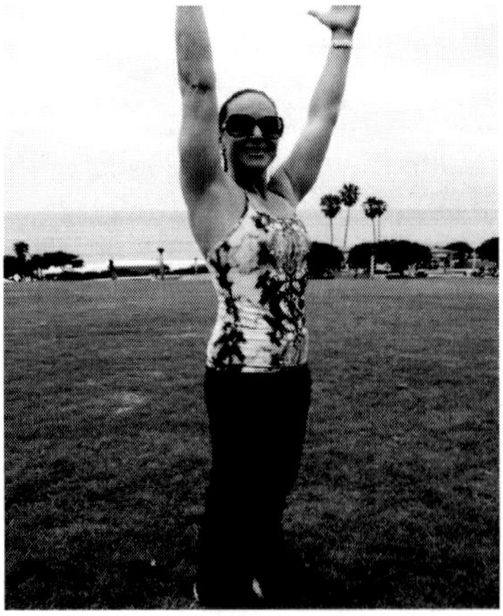

AVOIDING INJURY

Whenever you work out, or move for that matter, you always run the risk of injury. Now, there is no 100% fool-proof method out there for avoiding injury, but here are my top 10 ways that I've found to avoid injuries:

#1 - **Have a physical.** If you're new to working out or haven't seen the doctor for a few years, please go get yourself a physical. We're not getting any younger, and if you have a heart condition or some other physical ailment, you may need to modify your workouts. It never hurts to check, and it's the best way to make sure you know your limits and avoid hurting yourself.

#2 - **Gradually ramp it up.** Don't expect to start out doing 20 reps on the pull up bar or to be running 3 miles right off the bat if you have never done it before. Work your way up to it gradually. Don't worry. At the end of this book, I include workouts for all levels of fitness.

#3- **Don't forget to stretch!** Enough said on that one above.

#4 - **Wear the right footwear.** If you've been wearing the same sneakers for years, it's time for new ones. Get running shoes for running and workout shoes for cross training. Or find ones that work for both. Go to a good store and try on different models to see what works best for you.

#5 - **Clothing matters.** You need to get wicking clothes for comfort. A cotton T-shirt doesn't allow your skin to breathe and will cause you to overheat. Even if you can't spend a lot, Target and Wal-Mart have a nice selection. But what I'm really talking about here is a sports bra. Get a good one. Please! Basically if your breasts bounce, your breast fibers are tearing. And torn breast fibers DO NOT repair. They just stay torn, which is what contributes to saggy boobs. Gravity does enough of that, thank you.

#6 - **Cross Train.** Doing the same thing over and over again not only causes boredom in your brain, it also causes muscle boredom. Worse, it also contributes to overuse injuries. So do yourself a favor and cross train to avoid over-stressing certain muscle groups (All the workouts here are designed for cross training!).

#7 - **Drink Water.** Make sure you're drinking water as you workout. Everybody is different, but depending on your intensity, plan on 16 to 24 ounces during your workouts. And if you're out in the sun, plan on drinking a little more.

#8 - **Don't Workout on Empty.** Make sure you have some fuel before you go workout. It will give you the energy you need. Even if it's just an apple, give your body something to go on.

#9 - **Listen to Your Body.** Only you know what you can do. If it hurts, stop. If you feel like you're going to pass out, stop. Working out should never cause pain, faintness or light headedness. If you feel unwell, listen to your body and stop.

#10 - **Give Yourself a Day of Rest.** Even the most well-conditioned athletes don't train 7 days a week. Everybody, no matter the fitness level, needs at least one day a week to rest and repair. Otherwise you'll wear your body down and risk injury.

Putting It All Together

CARDIO

Cardio is an integral part of your fitness. There are lots of different guidelines out there. For basic fitness, it's recommended to do 30 minutes of moderate cardio five days a week or 20 minutes of vigorous or more intense cardio three times a week. You really don't need to do more unless you're training for a fitness event like a race or you're trying to lose weight.

The good news? You don't need to do the 20 to 30 minutes all at once (Although, personally, I find it easier to do one workout a day as opposed to two or more).

Sometimes it's really difficult to carve out 30 minutes at one time. If you're finding it hard to fit it all in, try to find 10 minutes three times a day where you can get your heart rate up and increase your breathing. You'll still get great results and your heart will thank you.

There are really two types of cardio: endurance and bursts.

Bursts are exactly what it sounds, short bursts of energy. They're also normally pretty intense as you're pushing yourself to your maximum exertion. Any type of sprinting or plyometrics (I'll show you plyometrics in the exercise breakdown section) are considered cardio bursts.

Over 40 Note - a plyometric can also be known as a plyo. Plyos are fast, energetic bursts of energy where you're working for short periods of time at your maximum ability. For example, stand up and raise your arms above your head. Jump up as high as you can 10 times in a row. That's a plyometric move.

Endurance is more about doing cardio over an extended period of time. Depending on your current activity level, endurance for you can mean anywhere from 10 minutes or more. However, endurance normally relates to doing a cardio activity such as running, biking, hiking, and swimming for 30 minutes and up. Brisk walking can also be included here.

Now, when you're working on improving your endurance or distance, you'll want to follow the long and slow theory. That's because you can't push yourself to work at your maximum heart rate for that long. Instead, you'll want to work out at 65-75% of your maximum capacity, or the fastest that you know that you can run. Otherwise, you'll burn out and won't be able to go the distance.

Think of it as pacing yourself. You don't want to sprint or go top speed when you go far; you just can't keep that kind of pace for long periods of time. Many coaches will have you base your effort on your actual heart rate. The best way to determine your exertion rate is to wear a heart rate monitor.

And if you can't afford a heart monitor or don't want to wear one, here's another option to try. When you're doing endurance training, you know you're going at the right pace when you can talk. I'm not saying you can hold a full on conversation (if you can, you're probably not working hard enough). It should take some extra effort to talk, but if you find you can't speak at all, back off the intensity until you can.

Now, when you are doing cardio bursts or plyos, you shouldn't be able to talk at all because you're working at your maximum intensity. So if you can, you're not working hard enough and you need to ramp it up.

While this isn't a total fool-proof method, it does work pretty well at keeping you in your target heart range.

Keep this in mind when doing any type of cardio workout. Whenever I have you doing a burst (sprint or plyo), work to your maximum. Try to talk. It should come out in ragged, breathless bursts. When you're doing more endurance work, you should be able to talk with just a little extra effort.

STRENGTH TRAINING

A lot of women aren't quite as familiar with strength training as they are with cardio. And let's face it: years ago, strength training was seen as more of a man's workout than for women. Women feared bulking up and there really wasn't anyone to show them the way.

But that's all in the past.

Strength training should be an integral part of your fitness routine. It helps build muscle mass and keeps your bones strong.

Considering that women are at a much greater risk for osteoporosis and osteopenia, why wouldn't you do it?

Contrary to the beliefs of the past, strength training (also known as resistance training) doesn't cause us to bulk up; it keeps us looking long and lean. Not to mention it has a wonderful side benefit: when you build muscle, you burn A LOT more calories. Even while you're at rest; just sitting around watching TV.

Let me explain. Yes it's true; a pound is a pound is a pound. A pound of fat may weigh the same as a pound of muscle, but that pound is in no way equal. That's because muscle is much denser than fat, so it makes you look leaner. But the best part? A pound of muscle burns about 50 calories a day. Fat burns a paltry two. Yes, you read that right. Just two calories. If that doesn't give you incentive to move it, I don't know what will. You can eat more! And still lose the weight. Bonus!

To get more out of your strength training, here are my five tips.

Tip #1 - **Avoid the machines.** If you're a gym gal, stay clear of the machines and head to the free weights. Weight machines tend to work on one isolated muscle. Plus, they typically have us moving in a way we don't typically move. Instead, use the free weights. You can replicate more functional exercises, plus they have the added benefit of incorporating more than one muscle in each move. Think about squats. A squat uses your whole lower body. Plus, it replicates how we should properly bend to pick up heavy items. Much better than a weight machine that just has you working on your gluteus maximus (aka your butt).

Tip #2 - **Intervals are the way to go.** In order to get the biggest bang for your buck, interval training is key. By interval training I mean mixing cardio in with your strength training. Why? By mixing the two together you'll keep your heart rate elevated, thereby increasing the calories you burn.

Tip #3 - **You need to feel it.** Don't think you can only lift 2 or 3 pound weights; the key to getting results is to make sure that you can actually feel the resistance. So don't be afraid to move up. That said, when you're doing intervals, you're going to use lighter weights. For my workouts, I recommend at least three pound weights but no more than five. If you don't feel like these are enough, you're not pushing yourself during the cardio portion enough or you're doing the reps way too fast.

Tip #4 - **Slow it down.** When you lift weights, I want you to really concentrate on the lowering of the weight. That's right, the lowering, or "negative" as it's called, causes an eccentric contraction. Don't worry about the term, just know that particular contraction is actually the most important part of the exercise. Eccentric contraction means muscle lengthening. I can't tell you how many times I see people lifting too fast. If you do it too fast, you're missing out on the resistance as you lower the weight which is more than half of the exercise!!!! So you're really doing yourself a disservice. The best way to make sure you're doing resistance training at a proper speed is to do it in two counts. Two counts up, two counts down. So in your head, count 1, 2 as you lift and then 1, 2 as you lower the weight or position. In other words, SLOW DOWN!!!

Tip #5 - **Don't be afraid to increase.** Some experts, such as Cosgrove, suggest letting the number of repetitions dictate how much weight you start with. Pick a weight that you can definitely lift 8 times, maybe 10, but certainly not more than 12 consecutive times. Ideally, you'd increase that weight a smidgen every time you do the routine, but since most weights come in 5-pound increments, he suggests this instead: Do 10 reps in a set the first time, then 11, then 12, and once you're doing sets of 12, increase the weight and go back to 10 reps per set. (His program calls for different numbers of sets, depending on the stage, but two to three sets for 10 to 12 reps is a good rule of thumb.)

THE CORE & MORE

WHAT IS THE "CORE"?

I'm sure you've heard the word "core." It's a word that gets tossed around a lot. That's because we finally understand that your core is really the center of your body's universe. Believe it or not, it's where all movement is generated. It helps you stand upright, keep your balance, it provides a stable base for exercise, and keeps your back protected. A strong core provides support for your whole body (and especially your spine), for just about any activity.

A strong core actually protects and strengthens your back, it supports your body so you sit taller, and it helps you alleviate the pressure on your joints. Using the core helps you utilize all of your muscles more efficiently and effectively. So don't think of it as just a way to get a flat belly; think of it as a way to get a longer, stronger, and meaner body for you!

In other words, it's a critical part of your body. The problem is, most of us don't necessarily train it. That's why it weakens and your joints start to take over. If you don't believe me, think of all the times that you sit over a computer or flop on the couch when watching TV; it's very likely you don't even think for an instant about pulling your belly in order to sit up straight. Pay attention to your posture and you'll start to realize how much you neglect this area.

If you have a weak core, you'll be more susceptible to poor posture, lower back pain, muscle injuries, and poor alignment throughout the body - all of which lead to muscle injuries. In fact, training your core will provide your body with the support it needs to help prevent pain and injury.

The concept of the core isn't new. Have you heard of Pilates? Pilates is a whole method of exercise that is based upon the premise of engaging the core to work the body from the inside out. In fact, Joe Pilates, creator of the Pilates method, pioneered the idea of the core over 80 years ago. But this also doesn't mean that the only way to strengthen your core is by Pilates. There are many different exercises that will help. Just know that by working and strengthening this area of your body will create a stronger, healthier you as well as allow you to boost your overall performance in both your fitness and daily life.

WHERE IS MY D%$# CORE ANYHOW?

Do you know how many women swear they don't have a core? Of course you do!!! Just because you're not sure where it is, or lost track of it, doesn't mean it you don't have one.

OK, let's investigate and find out exactly where it is. It's more than just your abs. Think of it as one big rectangle in the center of your body, going hip to hip, shoulder blade to shoulder blade, both front and back, all the way around.

That means the core is comprised of a wide variety muscles, with the majority located in the belly as well as the low and mid back. Twenty nine core muscles to be exact! It doesn't include the shoulders or any part of your neck. However, it does provide tremendous support to that area!

Front View: Shoulder to Shoulder & Hip to Hip

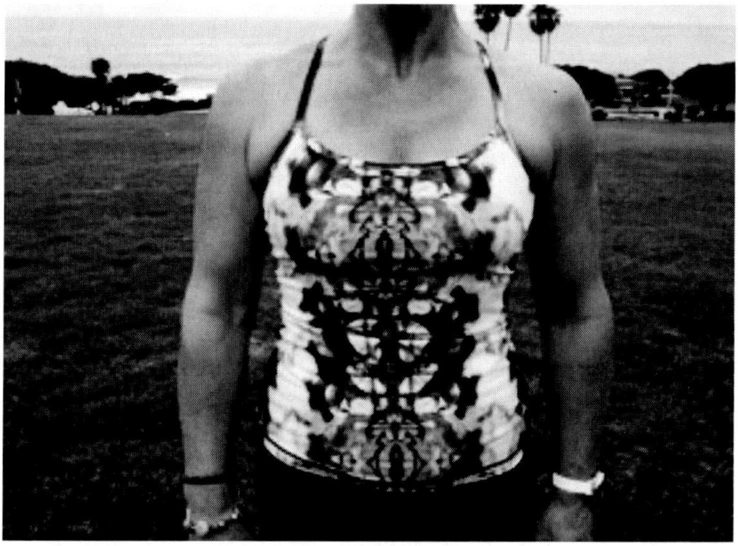

Rear View: Shoulder to Shoulder & Hip to Hip

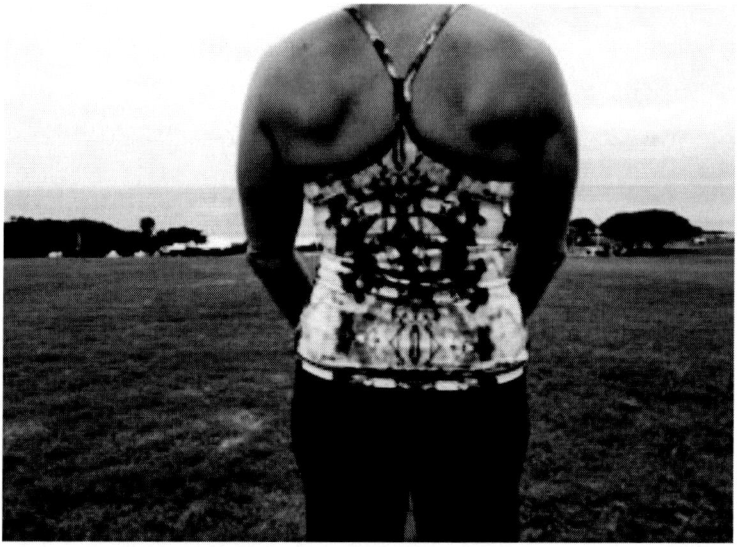

HOW TO STRENGTHEN YOUR CORE

Strengthening your core requires regular and proper exercise of your body's 29 core muscles. There's more to it than just doing a couple of traditional sit ups; that movement only works on the outer layer. True, when those muscles are worked you can get the look of six pack abs. Problem is, they don't really do much to strengthen your overall core.

Instead, the idea is to really focus on your form and focus on exercises that require you to engage multiple muscles at one time. That way, exercising 29 muscles doesn't seem so daunting either! Here are a few basic exercises that I recommend that just about anyone can do to enhance their core fitness:

- Bridge
- Abdominal crunch or sit-up
- Plank

This is not a comprehensive list by any means! It's just a few exercises to get you started. But more importantly, it's how you do them. A regular sit up isn't going to do much for your core. In fact, traditional abdominal exercises tend to work only the outer layer of abdominal muscles. Those are the muscles that when worked, give you the six pack abs. And while that looks really good, unfortunately, it doesn't really do much to strengthen your overall core and contribute to your overall fitness. Instead, change how you do your ab work and not only will you get a stronger core, but you'll still get sleek, sexy abs. Promise!

The Bridge:

Starting Position: arms at your side with your feet flat, hip distance apart.

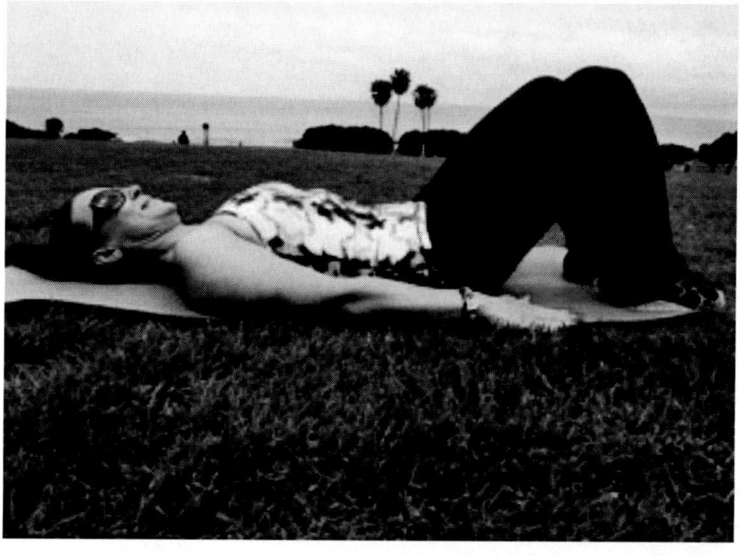

Slowly curl your hips and lift up towards the sky. Hold for a second, and then lower down.

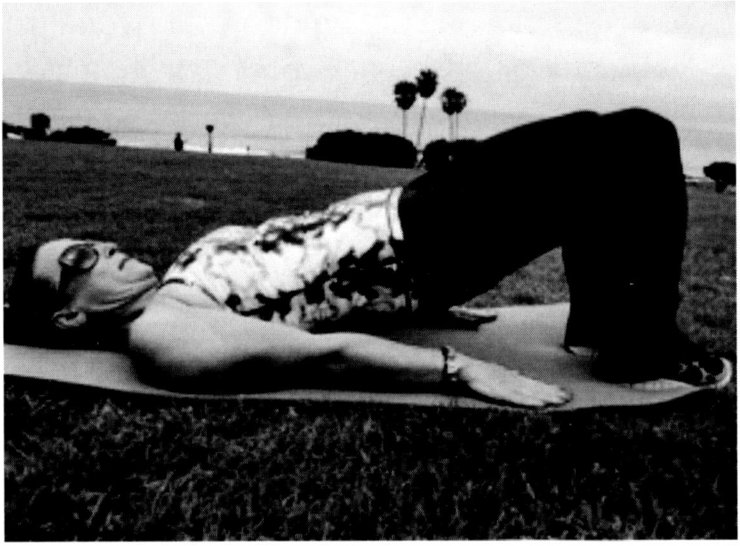

Abdominal Crunch:

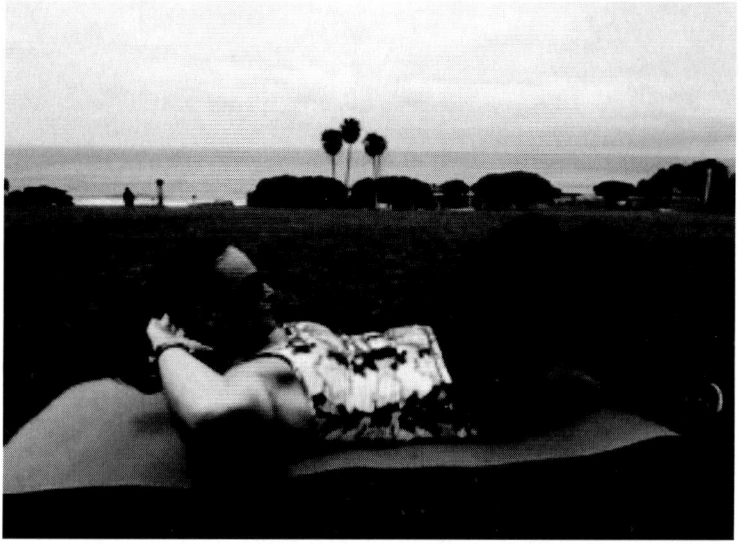

Plank:

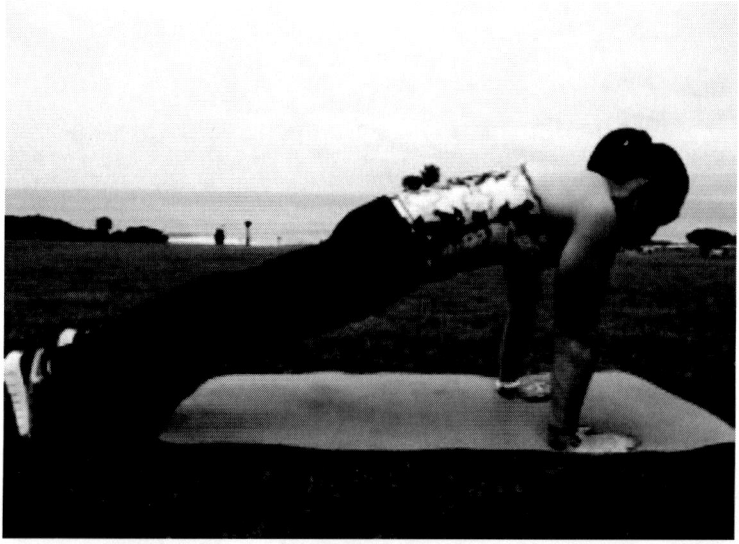

ENGAGING YOUR CORE

So, how do you engage multiple muscles? And what exactly is the right form? There are several things that you always need to think about and do when working on your core. The first is to engage starting from the bottom up, meaning your hips. Think about holding a continuous pelvic curl. This will engage your hips as well as your pelvic floor.

I know that this can be a hard idea for some people to understand. But it's really easy! Think about Kegel exercises. Yes, you read that correctly - the infamous Kegel.

If you don't know what a Kegel is, it's time to head to Google or your search engine of choice! This is a very important thing for any woman to know.

Before you run off to do them, please understand that it's not really about doing your Kegels here. It's more about holding that position, meaning essentially that you've tucked your tailbone under you and curled your hips up towards your navel. Believe it or not, by doing that you're going to be able to engage your lower core muscles, all the way up to your navel. This will drastically improve your abdominal strength.

Over 40 Note: It might not look like much, but this is an important concept to get. Why? Because the pelvic curl is also a basic position for many strength training moves. It strengthens your abs AND protects your back.

Pelvic Curl:

Neutral Starting Position:

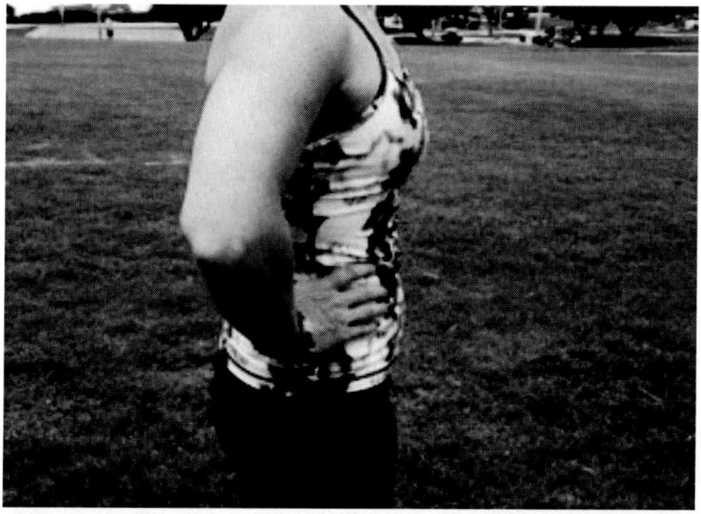

The Pelvic Curl In Action:

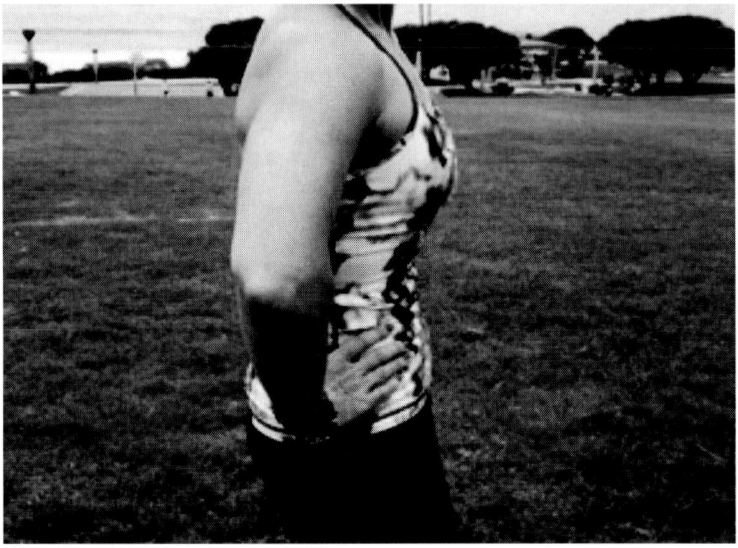

Moving on up the body, you get to what's known as your upper abdominals. It's that area right between, as well as behind, your rib cage. This is a hard area to train, don't be fooled. Take a second and try to engage it right now. Hard, right? And if you can't really feel it, how are you supposed to engage it?

One of the best ways that I've found for you to find that area in your own body is to simply think about your breathing. Normally, when we breathe, we breathe very shallow. In fact, most humans only use about 10% of their lung capacity. So take a deep breath and slowly let it release.

What happened to your rib cage? It started to protrude outwards as you took a breath, didn't it? Now, try it another way. You'll have to think a bit for this one! Take a deep breath and try to have your rib cage expand laterally, or out to the side, instead. I always find it helps to put your hands on the sides of your rib cage, just so you have a reference.

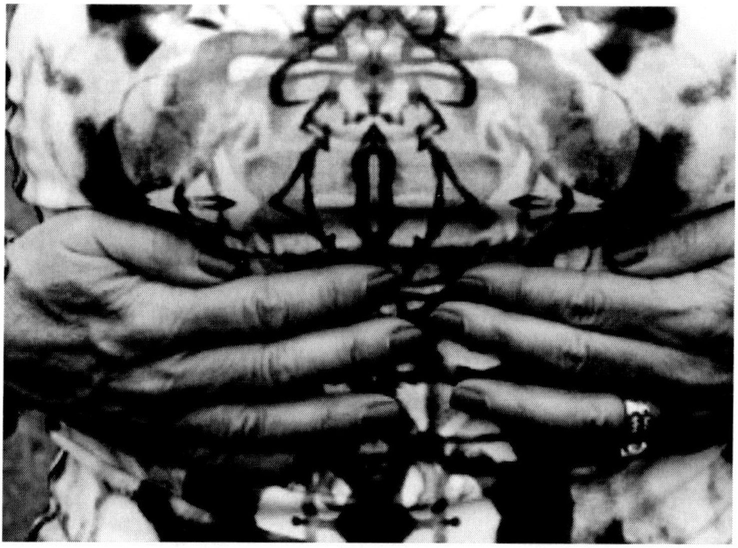

Try it again, thinking about expanding and contracting your rib cage out to the side. Those muscles you had to engage to do that are what help make up the upper part of your core. Trust me, with practice it does get easier!

Now, it's time to move around the body and focus on some of the muscles on your back, starting with the upper area around your shoulder blades. To engage this area, locate your shoulder blades and try to pull them down your back. But here's the tricky part: try not to let go of the other areas while you do this.

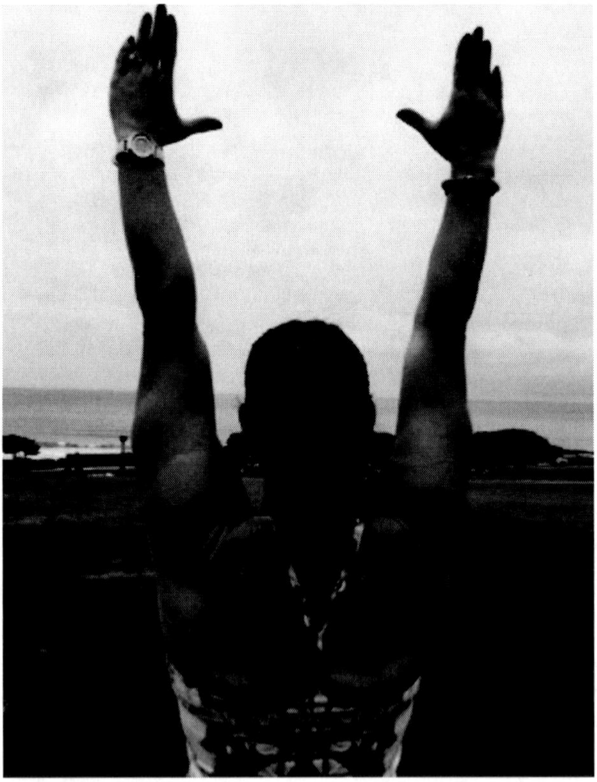

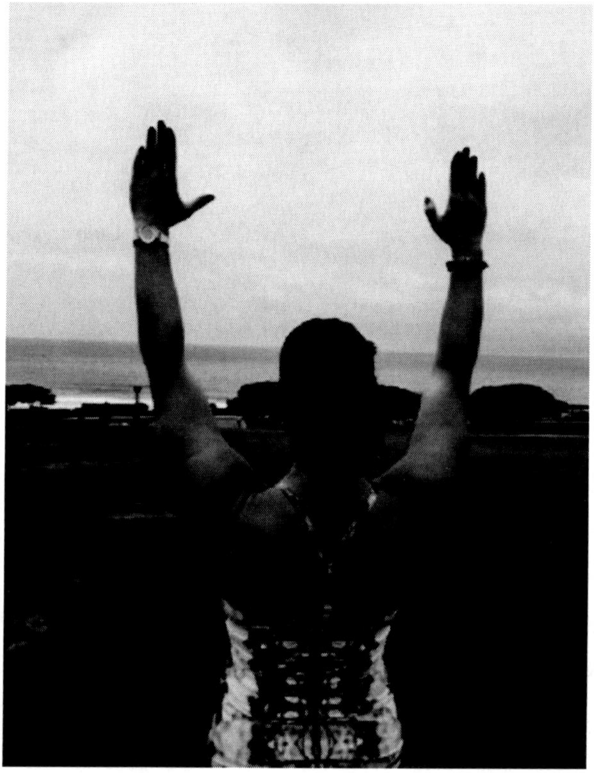

When you can pull your shoulder blades down and not move anything else, you're learning how to pull your core into itself. In the fitness world, it's what's known as the midline. You are basically pulling the body into itself, while all the while you're lengthening your body. It can be as hard as it sounds, and it is. However, you CAN master it, and doing this one simple exercise can go a long way in creating a stronger core.

I'VE GOT SPIRIT...IT'S MORE THAN JUST A HIGH SCHOOL CHEER

I'm a big believer that you can't get your sexy back just by exercise and diet alone. In fact, I truly believe if you really want to get your sexy back, you've got to incorporate the mind, the body AND your spirit.

This isn't something that often gets addressed in a workout system. But then, this isn't your ordinary workout program, is it? This is about getting your sexy back. And getting your sexy back is more than just about working out; it's about getting your mojo back. And the only way to really do that is to connect to yourself. Plus, I feel it's something really important.

The only way you're really going to get that inner sexy goddess back and be ready to flaunt your stuff to the world is by first taking care of your inner self. In all of my years as a fitness instructor working only with women, I KNOW it's an area that I think is often overlooked.

In fact, many people don't even think of spirituality when it comes to fitness. But I totally disagree.

Why? Because taking care of yourself means taking care of your entire being. In other words, the whole you. You have to feed, work and nurture all of it, which includes your mind, your body as well as your spirit.

Again, I know this isn't something that you'll find in a lot of workout systems. Most just focus on your diet and workouts. But focusing on all three elements is something that I believe is essential to your overall well-being, especially as you age. It's the final piece that will help you to truly find peace and happiness with your body both inside and out.

THE DIFFERENCE BETWEEN RELIGION & SPIRITUALITY

Before you read any further let's talk about the difference between religion and spirituality.

First off, I'm not going to address religion, ANY religion here in this book. Religion is a highly personal, and often highly charged, topic that goes well beyond the scope of this book. And this book is about getting your sexy back through health and wellness; this is definitely NOT a religious book.

However, it's still important to distinguish between religion and spirituality because it's confusing to a lot of people. And although one isn't better than another, they are two entirely different things. So here's my way of thinking that I use to give you a frame of reference as you continue going through this chapter.

First let me start off by stating, religion isn't spirituality and spirituality isn't religion. That doesn't mean that they are mutually exclusive by any means, just that they don't necessarily mean the same thing.

So let's understand what religion is first. Again, this can be a highly charged topic, so let's keep this high level.

There are lots of definitions of religion, but I'll use the latest from Wikipedia. According to Wikipedia, religion can be defined as an organized collection of belief systems, cultural systems, and world views that relate humanity to spirituality and, sometimes to moral values. Many religions have narratives, symbols, traditions and sacred histories that are intended to give meaning to life or to explain the origin of life or the Universe. From their ideas about the cosmos and human nature, they tend to derive morality, ethics, religious laws or a preferred lifestyle. According to some estimates, there are roughly 4,200 religions in the world.

4,200!!!

Now, spirituality can be a bit tougher to define, and it's harder to find a mutually agreed upon definition. But most sources agree that modern spirituality is the process of turning inward, connecting to yourself and the universe, finding your own individual path, and honoring who it is you really are.

To summarize, religion is the organized aspect that unites people with a common belief system. In other words, it teaches you a prescribed set of beliefs and provides guidelines to follow. It can, but not always, also serve as a vehicle to help people get in touch with their spirituality.

However, spirituality doesn't provide any kind of framework. There are no hard and fast rules, which is why some people are uncomfortable with it! Instead, it's all about being able to look internally and find the wisdom and connection not only to yourself, but to others and the universe as a whole.

Two entirely different things, but they do have a common theme. And that's connecting with something larger than ourselves. This is a beautiful, wonderful thing!

THE QUEST FOR SPIRIT

If you had told me how critical the three elements of mind, body and fitness were to my overall health when I was younger, I wouldn't have understood the concept at all. I mean, I knew the basic mechanics, but I didn't really understand them. In other words, I believed that I needed to work, study, and go to school to train my mind. I knew that I had to work out to gain muscle and stay in shape. And the only way to be “spiritual” was to go to services and follow my religion.

But I didn’t really get it.

If that’s all you do, you’re just doing what you’re supposed to do, not what really resonates with your soul.

There’s so much more to all of this than what I could have ever envisioned as a girl in my twenties and early thirties. See? There are some great things about being over 40!

As you get older you come to understand that just because you study something, it doesn’t mean actually you learn and retain anything. Just because you go through the motions of working out doesn’t mean that your body is in shape. And just because you go to worship services doesn’t necessarily mean that you’re working on your spirituality.

You have to find a connection with it in order to make it work and be effective.

Let me explain.

Think about a class you took, that you had to take either in high school or college, but you had no interest in for whatever reason. So you crammed for the tests and passed the exams, maybe even got an "A", but after the class was over, you couldn't remember a thing. Why? It was just total memorization. No learning or interaction took place.

How about all the times you started or planned to start an exercise program, only to work out without really making the commitment? You went through the motions, but didn't push yourself or try very hard. Maybe you didn't do it often enough to see any results.

Or if you're like me, remember all of the times that you went to a religious service but just let your mind wander to everywhere but there.

Do you relate to any of these examples? Come on! Be honest with yourself.

That's because you weren't really vested in the outcome.

And how is just going through the motions on any of these things really taking care of your well-being or helping your body and mind to move forward and evolve? The honest answer is that just going through the motions doesn't do a darn thing, except maybe make yourself feel better and say that you did something so you can check it off your list. You studied? Check! You worked out? Check! You went to church on Sunday? Check! Well, then you must be a very good girl.

Except now you know better, because it doesn't really work that way. If you want to reap the benefits of anything, you have to do the work. If you want to gain knowledge, you have to learn. If you want to be fit and strong, you have to eat right and do work outs that count on a regular basis. And if you want to become more connected with the world, others and yourself, you have to become more spiritually based.

I don't want to beat a dead horse and keep harping about nutrition and the importance of exercise. I know you get that or you wouldn't have read this far. And I know we all understand the importance of working our brains.

You know that those are things that you need to do in order to take care of yourselves and your body as you age.

But honestly, at the end of the day, working on your mind and body both take a back seat to working on your spirituality. It truly is the key to everything, including your hotness.

CONNECTING WITH YOUR SPIRITUALITY

Spirituality is all about looking inward and coming to understand the world and your place and role within it. Because it is such an intimate journey, everyone has their own unique path.

To me, spirituality is a very personal thing; far be it for me to tell you how to find it and incorporate it into your own world. And if it's already a part of your life, wonderful! If it isn't, all I can tell you is that it will change everything about you and your life for the better.

For some spirituality is about religion, for others it's not. Maybe it's a combination of both. That's up to you. The common element is connecting with something which is so much larger than our own interests.

My own personal journey has had many twists and turns. I grew up Catholic and it just never resonated with me. Trust me, we were not the casual church goers. I went to CCD (Catholic version of Sunday school) until I graduated high school. But I just personally never really got it; I'm a girl who needs to know the "why" of things, so belonging to a church where I wasn't allowed to question anything just didn't sit well with me.

I ended up leaving the church pretty much as soon as I went to college when my mother wasn't there to make me go to mass each and every Sunday morning. But that didn't feel right to me either, I felt like there was a hole in my life. I grew up in a home where religion was important, and to go from that to not having any religion wasn't what I wanted either. But I didn't know what else to do.

So after a lot of searching, I eventually ended up converting to Judaism in my mid-30s. That felt more right to me from a religious perspective. However, little did I know that was just the start of my journey. Converting had opened my eyes to all kinds of things and made me realize how much I didn't know or understand about religion and spirituality. So even after my conversion, I still felt I was on a spiritual quest. I kept looking and searching for more. And at the age of 40, I began embarking on some very personal internal reflection and started studying the laws of the universe with a very gifted teacher. I still study and learn to this day with all kinds of teachers. I'm still a work in progress, but I feel like I'm finally on the right path…and that works for me.

We each have our own story about who we are and what it is we are to become. Your path is going to be as unique and beautiful as you are. We have to stop judging each other and celebrate that we're all different. Being different is a good thing! Who wants a world of just vanilla? It's not that vanilla isn't wonderful. But if vanilla is all that you get, the world can be a very boring place.

We need to accept and respect the fact that all of us connect and learn in different ways. What works for you might not work for me and vice versa. As women, we need to celebrate our differences and understand that at the end of the day, we really all want the same things: peace, love and security for ourselves and our loved ones.

GETTING CONNECTED

To get started, or further your own spiritual growth, you need to take a moment to think about what spirituality means to you. Determine what role that you want it to play in your life, so you have a better idea of how to move forward.

In order to live spiritually, you need to stay connected, not only to yourself but to those around you in a very genuine way. Just like working out and eating right, it's a daily choice. Unfortunately, because you can't see it or touch it, because you don't always feel you need it to do your job, or you have 20 bazillion other things on your plate, it's an easy thing to push aside.

That's why you need to find ways to stay in touch with your own spirituality and spend time with people on a similar path. Surround yourself with good people in any way you can. Good people will always reinforce any good thoughts that you have. Thoughts truly become things - so why not fill your mind and heart with as many good ones as you can? There are a lot of great ways to connect with like-minded women. Depending upon your interests, try a church group, a spirituality class, or a group meditation. Search out classes in your town or find them online. There are lots of ways to connect with others! Then when you're at home, you may want to try using images, pictures, prayers, books, affirmations and meditation to remind yourself and help yourself tap into it whenever you can. I personally use all of these methods not all of the time, but yes, they are all tools that I rely on.

Why do I think you should embrace your spirituality? It gives you a sense of security in yourself and in the world. It really will help you feel happier and less stressed. And when you're happier, less stressed and feel more connected to yourself and to others, you're more inclined to take care of other aspects of your life such as nutrition and your body.

For me, my path to spirituality has given me a better perspective on the world, allowed me to forgive and grant grace to those around me, and remove people who are toxic and drain me of my energy. In the process, I've also learned to be a lot more gentle and forgiving to myself.

In other words, it's helped me become a better person, a better friend, and a better wife. It's encouraged me to take better care of my whole body. Why? I'm more at peace with myself. I feel much more secure and confident in my role and place in the world; overall, I have a better sense of me. Plus, because I take care of that part of my being, I'm more inclined to take care of the other parts of me as well ,because I want that feeling of happiness and contentment to spread to all aspects of my life.

Let your spirituality be a pillar of who you are and who you want to be. If it's a pillar in your life, it will always be there no matter what comes your way, or conversely, gets taken away. If you feel secure in yourself and the world that spirituality provides, you can handle whatever life throws your way. There is absolutely nothing you can't accomplish if your thoughts, actions and relationships are aligned with your vision of happiness.

When you're at peace with who you are and your life, your confidence and self-esteem soars. Then the real you can truly shine through.

And that is what true hotness really is.

TIPS ON FINDING YOUR ZEN

One of the best things that has improved my connection with my spirituality is meditation. Now before you go off and say I can't do that, or that I've tried it before and it didn't work, just know I used to say the same exact thing.

Here are all the excuses: My mind wanders; I can't sit still; It's a bunch of hooey; It does nothing for me; I just can't do it; Yadda yadda yadda.

I used to think all of that and more, because I used to believe that meditation meant just sitting there, trying to empty my brain and not think of anything for minutes on end. And no matter how much I tried and tried, my mind would inevitably wander. As a result, I felt like a failure and just took it as further proof that meditation wasn't for me.

But now I know better.

There are many ways to meditate which don't require sitting quiet in a dark room and emptying your mind of all thoughts. That can take years or a lifetime to learn! Who has time for that?

So here are some ways you can learn to successfully meditate and get your Zen on. This is by no means exhaustive, as there are as many ways to meditate as there are people in the world. You just have to find the one that works for you.

And don't be scared off by the word meditation or think it's some out there concept. It's actually been practiced for thousands of years and is gaining more and more acceptance in modern western medicine as a way to manage and reduce stress. So give it a try!

THE 5 MINUTE ZEN

Turns out, it only takes five minutes a day to get the full benefits of meditation. Five minutes! Plus, it's been scientifically proven that people who meditate are happier, healthier and more content with their lives.

And trust me, in those five minutes, your mind will wander. Except now you know that's OK and it's totally normal. It takes a lifetime of consistent practice to be able to let go of all thought. For most of us, that's just not going to happen. So instead, you're to simply acknowledge the thought, and then let it go.

I still have a hard time with that so I've found one of the best ways to keep me on track is to practice my breathing as a form of meditation. If this is your first try at meditating or you've experienced difficulty getting your mind to quiet down, here are the two exercises that I recommend.

Before you start, don't forget to set the timer for five minutes.

Option 1 - Taking deep, full breaths, count your breathing down from 100, with each inhale/exhale counting as one full breath. It's a very simple concept, and yes, your mind will still wander, especially around the halfway mark, but it's easier to stay on track when you're focused on your breathing; or

Option 2 - Breathe in for four counts through one nostril until your lungs can't take any more air, then exhale for four counts, exhaling out all of your breath through the other nostril. Stay focused on breathing in through one nostril for 10 full reps and then switch to the other nostril for breathing in. Keep changing the nostril you breathe in with after 10 counts until your five minutes are up.

I've personally used both of these methods and found that they both work because they give me something to focus and concentrate on. However, I personally prefer the second. It's actually a form of pranic breathing, which has some great health benefits such as improving your cardiovascular health and releasing your diaphragm.

I also like this method because not only do you have to count, you have to concentrate on filling and emptying your lungs. This means that you have to really concentrate on what you're doing, so your mind doesn't tend to wander as much. Not to mention, when you're done with your five minutes, you will feel great and supremely energized!

To practice this form of pranic breathing meditation, all you need to do is to extend either hand in front of your nose. Place your ring finger on one nostril and your thumb on the other to help you open and close the appropriate nostril. Set your timer and go. Simple!

THE NATURE ZEN

Who said you have to just be quiet in a room in your house to get your Zen on? That's crazy! If you're an outdoor girl, or even if you're not, try this method for a change of pace.

If spirituality is all about turning inward and connecting with others and all that is, what better place to do that than outside in nature? After all, where is it written that you have to sit still and quiet for it to be meditation? Meditation is about getting in touch with yourself.

Meditation can be as simple as walking outside and being still while you really hear the birds chirp, or standing at the beach smelling the salt air and watching the waves. It can be as easy as going on a nature hike and taking the time to smell the flowers.

Or maybe you just want to feel the sun truly warm your face and body.

Believe it or not, all of these are a form of meditating, because when you take the time to really listen, to really see and to really feel you HAVE to empty your mind of all other thoughts.

And that, my friend, is meditating.

The nature Zen is about getting yourself out there and really taking the time to feel and be one with nature. Spend five or ten minutes, or as much time as you need, to connect.

Because yes, when you do that, you are meditating!

THE GUIDED ZEN

Sometimes we all need a little help and meditation is no exception. That's why you sometimes need what's called the Guided Zen.

The guided Zen is a wonderful way to do meditation and one that I also personally use. It's where someone "guides" you through an actual meditation exercise using guided imagery or visualization.

This one is super if you have a real problem with quieting your mind, because someone is actually telling you what to do. Using all of your senses you are actually guided to relax, reflect, and de-stress.

These are typically a bit longer in length, with ten minutes normally being the minimum.

The key to this meditation is finding a teacher or guide whose meditation you enjoy listening to AND who helps you quiet your mind.

If you're already well along this journey, here's to getting more in touch with your spirituality. And if you're new, buckle up and get ready, it can be a wild ride. You're going to start learning things about yourself that you never knew. However, in reality, it's not that you didn't know, you just buried it deep inside. It's time to get in touch with who you really are!!

The Other Part of Sexy

So far, we've talked about many things including how to get started and establish a routine, nutrition, cardio, strength training, and even your spirituality. But I'm not done yet! There are a few more things to talk about before I share the workouts with you.

THE QUEST FOR SOME ZZZS

We all need an adequate amount of sleep. And while maybe you had trouble falling asleep here and there, it seems once you hit the big 4-0 you have trouble ALL THE TIME.

What's up with that?

Even if you can fall asleep it seems like any little thing will wake you up.

And if you've had a glass a water or cup of tea before bed? Forget about it! You know that you're going to have to get up to pee at least once if not twice.

Plus, once you're up, you're up. It can take a bit to fall back asleep.

Blame aging, blame hormones, and blame whatever you want. The end result is the same: you can't sleep!

So what's a gal to do???

First, it isn't just age. I won't deny that hormones probably play a part, but there's more to it than that.

Trust me; I know it's hard sometimes. When life comes at you from a million directions or your hormones are going crazy, or the kids and/or your significant other are going through trying times, it can be tough to get enough zzzs.

No one can really say what the right amount is, as it differs from person to person. I've seen amounts anywhere from 7 to 9 hours a day. Personally, I need my eight a night. You know for yourself what you really need.

Without getting enough sleep, your body doesn't get to recover from your workouts, nor does it get to recover from the stress of your day. Lack of sleep also causes our metabolism to slow down, ‘cause our minds start playing tricks on us (hallucinations), and we get really tired and cranky. Also, your muscles don't get time to recover and you feel sore and achy all over. End result? Lethargy, metabolism slow down and weight gain. No lie.

Now, if you’re one of the lucky gals who have never had a problem falling and staying asleep, you can stop reading right now. I’m quite envious of you.

But if you’re like me, and have started to find sleep a bit more elusive after the age of 40, you might want to keep on reading.

So what can you do to help you get the full-night’s rest that you really deserve and need? First, set a routine and follow it nightly. It can range from putting on your PJs to just getting ready for the next day. But do it at the same time every night. That way, it acts as a signal to your brain that it should be getting ready for sleep.

Two side notes:

First, don't use your computer, iPad, or even watch TV late at night. They'll stimulate you when you're really trying to wind down. You may need your nightly dose of the Nightly News, The Daily Show, or Leno, but you're not doing yourself any favors by watching that late at night. Personally, I DVR The Daily Show and watch it the next day.

Second, don't drink tea in the evening. Even chamomile. I know a lot of you drink tea to calm down and relax. Chamomile is a great one for that! But tea, any tea, also stimulates your bladder. Sad but true. So while it may help you fall asleep, it probably won't help you stay asleep, if you know what I mean.

Then, in your room, you'll want to keep it as dark as possible. It's all part of your body's natural biorhythms. Light stimulates and naturally encourages your body to be awake. Conversely, when it's dark, your body understands that it wants to sleep. If there is any light in your room, it can cause difficulty in both falling and staying asleep.

So pull down the shades and shut the door to block out any light. Remove as many electronics as you can. Try charging your phone, iPads, etc. somewhere else. Their light is brighter than you think and can cause you to wake up during the night. Plus, the emissions they put out, small as they are, can also disrupt your sleep.

You may also want to try an eye mask. I personally use one, as it really helps to block the light. It took me a bit to adjust, but I was amazed at how much better I slept with it on. I always wake up a whole lot less during the night when I wear one.

Lastly, make sure you go to bed and wake up at approximately the same time every day. I know we all like to sleep in on our weekends, but even then, try to stay within 30-60 minutes of your normal times. It really helps your body adjust to a schedule.

WHATCHA GOT ON UNDER THERE?

Let's get personal here shall we?

Because there is something that I have to ask, I really really do. And you might find it a bit personal, but after everything we've talked about so far, what's a little more, right?

It's time to discuss what's going on under your clothes. In particular, your bra.

When was the last time you had a bra fitting? A year or two ago? 10 years? Have you ever had a fitting???

If you've ever watched Oprah, then you know some of her most popular shows are the jean and bra makeovers. I'll get to the jeans in a bit, but let's focus on the bra first.

There are lots of numbers out there, but it's been said that up to 80% of American women are wearing the wrong size bra. And if you haven't had a bra fitting in the last year, then that probably means you.

Why is wearing the right size so important? Because wearing the proper bra is going to make you look about 10 pounds slimmer and do a whole heck of a lot for your self-esteem. You'll be amazed at how much better, taller, and slimmer you look just by just wearing the right size bra.

So if you haven't had a fitting you are doing yourself a real disservice. And if you think you're wearing the right size, let me give you my own little story. It's a little embarrassing. Heck, it's a LOT embarrassing. But it's also funny.

It also illustrates how way off base you can be with your sizing.

I personally had never had a bra fitting until about 5 years ago. Why would I want to do that? I can measure myself thank you! I don't need someone else to do it for me.

I looked up how to measure, followed the guidelines and measured both underneath and around my breasts.

According to all the guides, based on my measurements, I should wear a 36A.

Now, I know you don't know me, but I'm 5 feet 2 inches and while I don't necessarily have a small frame, I'm not a big girl. I also don't have a huge chest. But I always thought I was more than an A cup! However, if that's what the guides said, then that's what I should wear.

So I wore a 36A for I don't know how many years. And no matter what I did, the back would always ride up and the straps would always keep falling down.

Two signs, by the way, that your bra doesn't fit.

About five years ago, I was shopping at the big Nordstrom's sale in July for bras and underwear. I was lamenting to myself how few bras there were to choose from in my size when a nice sales lady asked me if I'd like a fitting. For some reason I said, "sure." I must have just seen the bra fitting show on Oprah or something. It really was something I kept meaning to do, but put it off, because who really wants to make time to have a bra fitting?

She asked me what size I wore and when I responded “36A” she took a quick look at my chest and very nicely said that she didn’t think so. At a minimum, I was a 34B. But it was more likely that I was more like a 32D.

I laughed. Seriously, me? A 32D? I wasn’t the one in my family with the big chest. Others, yes. But me? No way! I knew I had breasts, but a D? No offense, but isn’t a D cup huge?

Stay with me, we’re getting to the funny part.

But first, know that if you haven’t had a bra fitting, it’s really no big deal. It’s very discreet and no one touches or sees anything that you don’t want them to. Personally, I figure we both have breasts and she’s a professional, so what do I care?

Anyhow, I tried on my 36A for her and showed her how it fit. In fact, I think I even said something to the effect, “See? It fits.” She took one look at me and asked me what was hanging out the side of my bra. I said, “That? That’s just fat. I need to lose a couple of pounds.”

She started laughing at me (in a nice way) and said, “Oh no honey, that’s your breast.”

It was funny, but I felt like an idiot!

Who knew that ALL of it was supposed to fit in there? I’m not talking about front boobage, I’m talking about the sides too. I just thought I carried some extra weight there. Who knew that was also my breast???

Anyhow, she kept bringing bras back until we found the right size. When I tried it on, I just knew it. My girls were perky, I stood a little taller and I looked a whole lot slimmer. I knew I had found the right one at last.

When I asked the size, she said, “32D”. Who knew?

If I can be that far off not just in size, but also how a bra is supposed to fit, then chances are you are too. So go get a bra fitting. Go to a bra store, go to a large department store or go to Victoria’s Secret. They can honestly help you. You’ll find the size and style that works best for you. Plus, it’s pain free and you’ll look like you dropped 10 pounds.

For most of us, our moms buy our bras when we're preteens and/or teens, and then we just sort of hang around that number. At that age, it's not like you let your mom see anything. And just think, no one probably told her about or explained a bra fitting to her either, so how could she know exactly how a bra should fit and be able to pass that info on to you?

Now before I finish this topic, one last note. You're supposed to get a bra fitting every 6 months. Well, that's probably not going to happen. But try to go at least once a year or every other year. Your breasts change with your weight, hormones and age. I know mine just did and sure enough, I had to go up another cup size.

So go get a bra fitting. This one simple thing will go a long way to getting your sexy back.

And, by the way, pick up some pretty undies while you're there too.

MAKING YOURSELF A PRIORITY

If there is one thing that most women are bad at, that's carving out time for ourselves, or often, even spending money on ourselves. We tend to give to everyone else and always put ourselves at the back of the pack.

That's got to end; you just can't keep putting yourself last.

Why? Just honestly ask yourself the following, "If I keep putting myself last, then why should anyone ever put me first?"

Think about that one for a moment.

The fact is, if you don't place a priority on yourself from time to time, you can't expect anyone else to do it for you either. Be it your spouse, your kids, your friends, your boss, or your coworkers; they won't do it unless you do it first. And if you have a daughter this is extra important. **YOU** have to set the example.

This isn't about being selfish. This is about taking care of you and nourishing the woman who lives inside of you that wants, or really needs, to feel pretty, sexy, and desirable. She's not dead, she's just waiting to come out!!!

Trust me; I know that your money has to spread around to many things such as mortgages, cars, bills, food, clothes, gas, tuition etc. But for a lot of woman, it seems as though they put everything that everyone else needs on the budget except themselves.

But what about you? What do you need? It's really OK to spend some of that money on yourself. You need things too.

It's wonderful to be a kind, giving, loving person to the people around you. It truly is. But why does that mean that you can't be kind, giving and loving to yourself?

Don't hear me wrong. This isn't about squandering money you don't have by any means. But this is about placing equal importance on yourself.

After all, taking care of yourself makes you feel good about yourself, it makes you feel happy. And when you feel happy, you're more likely to show your happy self and spread the happy around to everyone else.

Plus, who doesn't like being and feeling happy?

When was the last time you went to a makeup counter and had your make up done with the latest colors? Then actually, gasp, bought some?

When was the last time you went to a good hair salon and had your hair professionally cut, colored and styled?

When was the last time you actually shopped for a pair of jeans that made you feel good and showed off your assets? Or a blouse that made you feel pretty?

Or maybe got a mani/pedi? Or even a bottle of fun polish?

Nails and make up not your thing? Then how about a massage that made you feel relaxed and peaceful?

By the way, notice how I didn't ask if hair wasn't your thing? If it's not, too bad. That's because we ALL need to take care of our hair. After 40, the natural look really is not a good option. This isn't about low/high maintenance; gray ages you, plain and simple. Unless you are one of the genetic few that has beautiful gray hair, of course. But even that doesn't excuse you from getting a good haircut though.

This isn't about being superficial. In fact, I don't think this is superficial at all. This is about finding ways to make yourself feel modern, relevant, pretty and dare I say, sexy!

We all know that we're not supposed to judge a book by its cover, but in reality we all do that. We're all guilty of making snap judgments about someone based on their looks occasionally. For example, think about the last time you saw a person who is dressed in a way that made you cross the street. That's a classic example of judging a book by its cover.

It's just part of human nature.

So let me ask, what kind of message do you think it sends to the world if you are only seen in faded baggy jeans, old shoes, and a baggy shirt with your hair back in a ponytail? Does that give the impression of a confident sexy woman? Does wearing clothes like that make you ***feel*** like a confident sexy woman?

I'm not saying that you need to look perfect all the time. I can't even imagine the pressure if we have to live up to that standard! But this is about giving yourself permission to spend a little money on yourself so you can feel like you're pretty. It doesn't have to be an overhaul, but find the things that make you feel like an attractive, desirable woman, because it really is OK to spend some money on yourself.

More than just giving yourself permission to do things to feel better about your outside appearance, it's also important that you set time aside for yourself so that you actually have the energy to give to everyone else.

So find a way to make time for yourself to do something you enjoy. Purchasing this book is a great start, but there has to be more. We all need to take some time off to pursue things that are of interest to us, even if it's just going to Starbucks for a coffee and reading the paper for 10 minutes in relative peace.

When you make time for yourself, you'll find your stress decreases. You're much more capable of dealing with the day to day grind. Not to mention, you'll find that when you give to yourself, you'll be much better at giving to others.

So stop placing yourself last.

I could add some words about stress, but frankly, if you are eating right, working out, growing spiritually, getting enough sleep and taking some time out for yourself, you're going to automatically find that you're better able to deal with the stress that comes your way.

The Workouts

*** Please consult a physician before starting any new workout program ***

The Over 40 and Still Hot Workouts are based on the principal of interval training. Interval means mixing high intensity with low intensity so each workout will include a mix of cardio to get your heart rate up along with strength training.

Trust me, there's a reason for this!

I gave you the story earlier about my first marathon. Well, when you train for a marathon you have to run - a lot. And we all know that cardio burns calories. So you would think that I lost a lot of weight while I was training to for a 26.2 mile race. Wrong!

I think I lost maybe a pound. Sure my hips, thighs, butt and calves got tighter. But the rest of me? Well, it wasn't a pretty look. Especially for a gal who already is prone to the apple shape with muscular legs.

But I digress.

There are two reasons why I only lost a pound. The first is because when you do a lot of cardio like that, you're burning a lot of calories. Plus, you're also building muscles, which in turn makes you get really hungry! So what do you do? You eat. And you tend to eat a lot because you think you deserve to. You even rationalize it by saying to yourself, "I worked out, I deserve it." Or worse, "I'll just run some more tomorrow." But of course, I never deserved as much as I thought I did!

The second reason is because I plateaued. See, when I was training, I was always running long distance and I always ran at about the same speed. My body acclimated and got used to the routine. Once that happened, my body became more efficient and didn't have to work nearly as hard as it did in the beginning. In turn, I wasn't creating any additional muscle; because I wasn't creating as much muscle after a certain point, I wasn't increasing my caloric burning rate. Rather, I was decreasing it. But I was still eating like crazy because mentally I thought that I could.

Luckily, I got turned on to interval training in my 30s. I've used interval training on my clients for years and does it work! It keeps both your mind and your body from getting bored. You're constantly mixing it up so it never knows what comes next. That way you continually build muscle, and because you're keeping your heart rate up, you're burning more calories. In a nutshell, mixing strength and cardio together really boosts the metabolism for the maximum caloric burning rate so you see results in less time.

There is one term that I want you to become familiar with and that's "reps." You may or may not know what that means. Reps is short for repetitions. Whenever you see or hear the word reps, you'll know that's how many times I want you to repeat that particular move at that time. For example, if you see bicep curls for 10 reps, that means I want you to do a bicep curl 10 times. You may also see that terminology used for cardio and plyometric moves.

For the most part, I do things by time. Meaning we do exercises for a specific period of time and you do as many as you can, without straining or stressing your body too much. You may want to keep a pad of paper next to you in the beginning to keep track of how many reps you do of a particular exercise. That way, you'll be able to track your progress.

I recommend that you do interval training at least 3 times a week. Five times is even better! However, if you haven't worked out for some time, if ever, you may find that five days of interval training is just too much. That's OK. For you, I want you to start at 3 days a week of interval training. For the other two days, you can do one of the add-on workouts or take a 20 to 30 minute brisk walk. Note the word brisk. I'm not talking about the weather; I'm talking about your speed. It's a gradual process. If you meet your body where it is, and don't try to do too much too soon, you'll find that you'll be up to a full five day interval workout training in no time.

This is a progressive program. So no matter what level of fitness you're currently at, don't do more than you feel comfortable with. Trust me, interval workouts are harder than they seem. Since your goal is to be working out five days per week, you'll want to make sure you're able to stick with it.

Please remember to go at your own pace, take breaks when needed, drink water throughout, and most of all have fun!!!

For a description of more of the moves/lifts, please refer to our website http://www.Over40andStillHot.com.

The Workout

Warm Up:

Alternating Knee Lifts (20 per leg)
Alternating Knee Lifts with Arms Overhead (20 per leg)
Alternating Knee Lifts with Twist (20 per leg)
Jog in place (20 reps)
Wide jog in place (20 reps)
Jog in place (20 reps)
Stationary Hip Opener (6 per leg)
Stationary Twist (10 reps)
Stationary Arm Circles (10 reps per arm each direction)

The Exercises (i.e. The Work):

Part 1: *All exercises are for 45 seconds followed by 15 seconds of rest. Use a timer.*

1. Jumping Jacks
2. Push Ups
3. Low Jumping Jacks
4. Right leg lunge with side shoulder lifts
5. Toe Jumps
6. Left leg lung with front shoulder lifts
7. Squat Jumps
8. Squat with shoulder press
9. High Knee Jog
10. Bicep Curls
11. Forward Toe Touches
12. Plie Squat with Pull Down
13. Mountain Climbers
14. Tricep Dip

Abdominals:
All abdominals are 12 reps each.

- Curls
- Hold Curl
- Pulse Curl
- Toe Raises
- Side Curl LEFT

- Side Curl Left Pulse
- Side Curl Left
- Side Curl Left Pulse
- Center Curl
- Hold Curl
- Pulse Curl
- Toe Raises
- Side Curl RIGHT
- Side Curl Right Pulse
- Side Curl Right
- Side Curl Right Pulse
- Center Bicycle

At this point, to continue the workout go to Part 2, otherwise, skip to the stretches.

Part 2:

Same as part 1, with the addition of 2 new exercises.

15. Jumping Jacks
16. Push Ups
17. Low Jumping Jacks
18. Side Steps
19. Toe Jumps
20. Right leg lunge with side shoulder lifts
21. Squat Jumps
22. Left leg lung with front shoulder lifts
23. High Knee Jog
24. Squat with shoulder press
25. Forward Toe Touches
26. Bicep Curls
27. Side Hops w/ optional Knee Touch
28. Plie Squat with Pull Down
29. Mountain Climbers
30. Tricep Dip

The Stretches (Otherwise known as the reward!!!)

Hold each stretch for a **minimum** of 20 seconds.

Calf Stretch with Shoulder Crossover Stretch (both sides)
Thigh (Quad) Stretch
Hip (Figure Four) Stretch
Hamstring Stretch
Back Round Up
Upper Back Round Stretch
Arm Press Stretch

Setting My Fitness Goals Worksheet

- What areas of my fitness am I most happy with?

- What area of my fitness would I like to see the most improvement? List them all.

- What are the top two areas that I would like to work on first?

- What goal can I set for myself to prove TO MYSELF that I have improved?

- What am I willing to do to get there?

- What are you willing to give up in order to meet your goals?

Congratulations!

You now have the start of a plan!!!

For a printable version, please go to

www.Over40StillHot.com/resources

Recommended Foods

This is just a guideline, and not meant to be all inclusive. Nor is it meant to replace the USDA recommended guidelines. This is just a simplified version for reference purposed only. To get a diet plan customized for your specific nutritional needs, please consult a physician or qualified nutritionist.

In addition to this chart, there are a couple of bonus foods to mention as well, such as beans, milk and avocados. They are both a carb AND a protein.

One final note, try to eat a meal consisting of a protein and a carb within 90 minutes of working out. You'll need them both for recovery.

Proteins 2-3 Servings per Day

Eggs or Egg Whites
Ground Chicken Breast
Ground Turkey Breast
Lean Ground Beef- 90% or more
Skinless Chicken Breast
Skinless Turkey Breast
Cottage Cheese
Low Fat Cheddar Cheese
Haddock
Mussels
Oysters
Salmon
Shrimp
Crab
Trout
Tuna - canned or fresh
Peanut Butter
Almond Butter
Almonds
Walnuts

Carbohydrates 6-11 Servings Per Day

Apples
Baked Potato - with skin
Baked Sweet Potato - with skin
Bananas
Barley
Blueberries
Cherries
Corn
Fat Free Yogurt
Oatmeal
Oranges
Raspberries
Squash
Strawberries
Tomatoes
Whole Grain Breads
Whole Wheat Pastas
Yams

Vegetables 3-5 Servings Per Day
Artichokes
Asparagus
Beets
Broccoli
Brussel Sprouts
Cabbage
Carrots
Cauliflower
Celery
Cucumbers
Dark green lettuces
Green Beans
Kale
Mushrooms
Onions
Peas
Peppers
Spinach
Squash
Tomatoes

FOOD DIARY

AS A GENERAL RULE OF THUMB, THE FOLLOWING IS A GUIDELINE OF THE DAILY REQUIRED SERVINGS.

Carbohydrates (6-11 Servings) Bread/Cereal/ Rice/Pasta

Fruits (2-4 Servings)

Veggies (3-5 Servings)

Proteins (2-3 Servings) Meat/Fish/Beans/Eggs/ Nuts

Dairy (2-4 Servings) Milk/Yogurt/Cheese/

Fats (Sparingly) Butter/Oils

Water (8-8 oz servings or more depending upon your weight)

The following page gives you an outline to easily track your progress. Please make additional copies as needed!

TODAY'S DATE:

LIST WHAT YOU ATE AT EACH MEAL.....MAKE SURE YOU LIST EVERYTHING!!!

BREAKFAST:

LUNCH:

DINNER:

SNACK:

SNACK:

TIMES I DRANK WATER:

TALLY IT UP!

OF CARB SERVINGS: _____
OF FRUIT SERVINGS: _____
OF VEGGIE SERVINGS: _____
OF PROTEIN SERVINGS: _____
OF DAIRY SERVINGS: _____
OF FATS: _____
GLASSES OF WATER: _____

Thank You!

COULD I ASK YOU FOR A FAVOR?

I see you've made it all the way to the end of my book Over 40 and Still Hot. I'm so glad you enjoyed it enough to get all the way through! If you liked the book, would you be open to take a minute or two and leaving me a 4 or 5 star review?You see, I'm a self published author, and when people like you are able to give me reviews, it helps me out in a big way. You can leave a review for me right here: **http://bit.ly/1ao1rKA**

It would really mean a lot to me.

Thank you,
Debby

About Debby

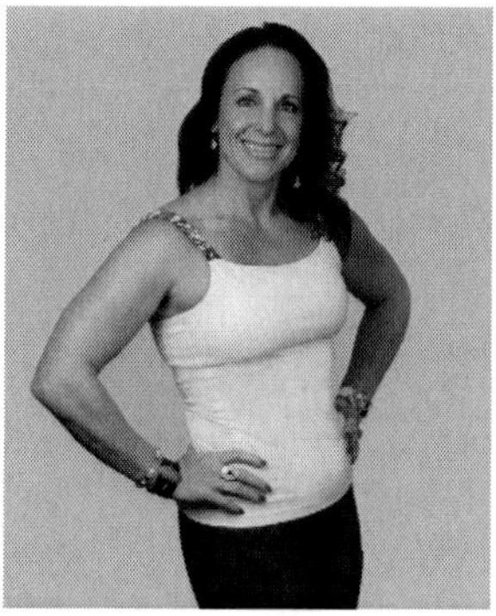

Debby Dowling is the owner and creator of the Over 40 and Still Hot fitness system. She's been involved with teaching women's fitness for the past 6 years. With a primary focus on women, Debby noticed that somewhere around the age of 40, women started feeling a little lost in their looks and a little more insecure with their bodies.

But she knew that it doesn't have to be that way! She believes that there really is a fountain of youth out there that you can claim. It's all about eating right, exercising, learning to love who you are and making yourself a priority.

Debby is a certified Adventure Boot Camp Instructor, AFAA Group Fitness Instructor, AFFA TeleFitness, NESTA Sports Nutritionist, Michael Miller Pilates Instructor and is certified in CPR. She is also a Reiki Master and Karuna Reiki Master.

Debby started and ran a very successful women's boot camp in La Grange, IL until moving to Southern California in early 2010. She now devotes her time to sharing what she knows with women around the world to help them get their sexy back.

Debby is living her dream along with her husband and three rescue doggies, all of whom are the loves of her life, by the beach in Dana Point, CA.

You can learn more about Debby and purchase the **Over 40 and Still Hot** fitness system **here**. Or visit **www.Over40StillHot.com** for more information and products.

Made in United States
North Haven, CT
10 November 2026

22096542R00098